Low Back Pain

A COLOUR ATLAS OF
LOW BACK PAIN

KENNETH MILLS
MA, BSc, FRCS
Consultant Orthopaedic Surgeon
Grampian Health Board, Aberdeen, Scotland.

GRAHAM PAGE
ChM, FRCS, MB, ChB
Consultant in Accident and Emergency Care
Grampian Health Board, Aberdeen, Scotland.

RICHARD SIWEK
FRPS, AIMBI
Assistant Director of Medical Illustration
University of Aberdeen

Wolfe Medical Publications Ltd

Copyright © Kenneth Mills, Graham Page, Richard Siwek, 1990
Published by Wolfe Medical Publications Ltd, 1990
Printed by W.S. Cowell Ltd, Ipswich, England
ISBN 0 7234 0959 5

A CIP catalogue record for this book is available from the British Library.

This book is one of the titles in the series of Wolfe Medical Atlases, a series that brings together the world's largest systematic published collection of diagnostic colour photographs.

For a full list of Atlases in the series, plus forthcoming titles and details of our surgical, dental and veterinary Atlases, please write to Wolfe Medical Publications Ltd, 2-16 Torrington Place, London WC1E 7LT, England.

Contents

Acknowledgements

We are grateful to Professor W. H. Kirkaldy-Willis, Emeritus Professor, Department of Orthopaedic Surgery, Saskatoon, Canada and Messrs Churchill Livingstone, New York for their permission to reproduce Figures **134** to **138** inclusive, from their book *Managing Low Back Pain*, 2nd Edition.

We acknowledge the help given to us by Miss Sarah Bertram, Miss Laura Garden, Mrs Moira Mills, Mrs Ann Preston, Mr Keith Mutch, Senior Medical Artist, Miss Libby Brand and Mrs Susan Strelley, Superintendent-Physiotherapists, Dr Alexander McDonald and Dr Frank Smith, Consultant Radiologists, Mr Douglas Wardlaw, Consultant Orthopaedic Surgeon, Mr Richard Morton, Director, Graves Medical Audiovisual Library, Chelmsford, Essex, Dr Stuart Denholm, Dr Alan McPherson and Dr Calum McLeod, Senior House Officers, Aberdeen Royal Infirmary.

We are also grateful to Dr Martin Roland, Cambridge and Messrs J.G. Lippincott, Philadelphia, for their kind permission to reproduce the questionnaire and diagram on low back pain on pages 18 and 19.

Preface

This is a short colour atlas about low back pain, that ubiquitous human complaint. Its aim is to present a logical approach to the diagnosis proceeding from a history to physical examination and to investigations. Emphasis is placed on the examination, because this is a feature often not well performed by physicians. Common non-invasive methods of treatment are illustrated and sophisticated methods of investigation and invasive treatment, including surgery, are mentioned.

The atlas is intended specifically for medical and paramedical personnel. The presentation is the product of a few individual attitudes. The authors are well aware that there are many other approaches to the problem of low back pain.

Low back pain

Low back pain is exceedingly common. Almost everyone over 40 years of age has had some serious episode of low back pain. Despite the personal and social consequences of such widespread disability, the accurate diagnosis and treatment of low back pain remain uncertain.

The combination of multiple joints in the lumbar spine (exposed to severe mechanical strains throughout life) with the end of the spinal cord and the cauda equina, makes precise localisation of pain production very difficult. To compound the difficulties pathology in the abdomen can often be expressed by low back pain.

A very wide range of congenital and acquired conditions can lead to lumbar backache, consequently the diagnosis of low back pain remains a grey area and a fertile ground for untrained manipulators, bone setters and faith healers. Accurate scientific research is badly needed to elucidate the localised causes of back ache—and these may be at several levels in any one individual. One of the difficulties is that only man has a vertical spinal column, so that animal models for investigation are unavailable.

In the past 10 years, the developments of computerised axial tomography (CT) and nuclear magnetic resonance imaging (NMRI) have revealed the detailed anatomy of the lumbar spine in a way that has never been possible with conventional radiography.

In considering the diagnosis for a patient with low back pain it is useful to think of three categories of pain production, i.e. the musculoskeletal system, the central and peripheral nervous system and the viscera. The history taking, physical examination and investigations can be directed to these three areas, thus ensuring that no serious or dangerous cause of back ache is overlooked.

The most effective manner of physical examination is to have the patient stripped down to his or her underclothes and to examine the patient first standing, then sitting and finally lying down. This progression causes least disturbance of those in severe pain. In each posture the examination can proceed from the trunk distally encompassing the body systems likely to be abnormal. Where pathology is discussed or illustrated, we have used the order of congenital, traumatic, infective, vascular, degenerative, neoplastic and biochemical causes.

Some causes of low back pain

These are listed in the order of congenital, traumatic, infective, vascular, visceral, degenerative, neoplastic, biochemical and psychological causes.

The most common are traumatic causes in the young and degenerative causes in the elderly. The other causes can be quite rare, but a comment about frequency is present in each section.

Spina bifida

Spina bifida occulta is not a common cause of low back pain and may not have any external manifestation. It arises from a failure of fusion of the neural and skeletal elements of the spine in early embryonic life. The more severe form gives rise to external myelomeningocoele and paraplegia. The occult form may present in childhood or early adult life with low back pain, with or without slow, progressive neurological deficits of varying types. There may be a midline skin dimple in the lumbosacral region, perhaps with surrounding pigmentation or hair. A motor defect may lead to asymmetry of leg length and shape, while a sensory defect may give rise to unnoticed injuries or ulceration.

Radiographs will show variable lack of fusion of the neural arches at one or two lower lumbar levels. There may be abnormalities in the posterior joint facets and transverse processes. The spinous processes are commonly absent. Such skeletal changes predispose to the development of back pain, perhaps precipitated by minor injury. Treatment is along conservative lines—analgesics, physiotherapy, splintage. If a progressive neurological deficit is present, investigations such as myelography or CT or NMR scans may lead to a neurosurgical exploration. This will relieve nerve root tension or pressure but if further bone loss is produced, a local spinal fusion may be necessary.

Scoliosis

Scoliosis is a curvature of the spine in the coronal plane. It is termed 'primary' if the vertebrae are changed in shape. It is usually painless until degenerative changes occur in middle age. It may be congenital from malformation of the vertebral bodies or neural arches. Such curvature may increase with growth and may not be compensated by secondary curves in the opposite direction. Congenital scoliosis may eventually lead to partial paralysis in the adolescent period in the levels distal to the curve.

Scoliosis after injury and infection is rare. Kyphosis is much more common. In the western world, scoliosis stemming from neuromuscular causes is becoming rare with the falling incidence of poliomyelitis and the muscular dystrophies. However, minor curvatures resulting from degeneration of the spinal joints with or without osteoporosis compressions are increasing.

So-called idiopathic scoliosis, for which no cause can be found, is a deformity of adolescents, particularly girls. It can progress rapidly from normality to gross deformity in 1-2 years. No distal paralysis develops.

Infantile scoliosis is a temporary curvature resulting from the baby lying constantly on one side, while the skeleton is very young and soft. It is associated with plagiocephaly but both deformities usually resolve spontaneously.

A secondary scoliosis is a curvature caused by a short leg or a disc prolapse, etc. When the patient is horizontal, the spine will straighten.

Primary scolioses are nearly always linked to an element of vertebral rotation; in the growing skeleton this leads to a rib hump deformity on the convex side of the thoracic curve. To keep balanced with the head above the pelvis, the spine develops compensatory curves above and below the primary curve. After the third decade of life, degenerative changes develop above and below the primary curve.

Symptoms from scoliosis are absent at first. Usually the parents of the child first notice the asymmetry when one shoulder appears higher than the other or one hip appears more prominent. Clothes do not fit properly and soon there is distortion of the rib cage. The range of spinal movements is reduced but without pain. A neurological deficit may be present if poliomyelitis neurofibromatosis or a muscular dystrophy is the underlying cause. As degenerative changes develop, so the range of spinal movement is reduced and pain on movement slowly worsens.

Treatment is concentrated on the early changes to prevent progression of the curve (braces and jackets). If this fails, a long spinal fusion is required after the age of 12-14 years. The pain of degenerative changes can be palliated by physiotherapy and partly controlled by a brace or a corset.

Spondylolisthesis

This condition is defined as the shift of one vertebral body on the one beneath in the sagittal plane. By far the most common shift is forwards; a backward shift is rare and is caused by degenerative changes (retro-spondylolisthesis). Whichever the direction of the shift, spondylolisthesis is not a common cause of low back pain.

There are a number of causes. The pars intra-articularis of the neural arch may be lengthened by congenital malformation of the facets or by soft bones (osteogenesis imperfecta). This is rare. The pars intra-articularis may be fractured on one or both sides by major violence or by repeated stress. In the past the fatigue fractures were thought to result from failure of fusion of ossific centres of the infantile neural arch, because this type is most often seen in adolescence. Finally, the articular cartilage of the posterior facetal joints may degenerate sufficiently to allow a small forward shift. This is not progressive whereas the other forms of spondylolisthesis may allow a slow steady displacement, so that in the most gross forms the upper vertebral body may lie totally anterior to the lower vertebral body at the same level.

In the lumbar region the L4/5 level is most often affected by degenerative spondylolisthesis, while the L5/S1 level is most often affected by trauma. However, any level can be affected. Low back pain is the chief symptom. This begins gradually and intermittently but becomes severe and unremitting and is worsened by movement. In the traumatic variety (often occurring in adolescence), the nerve roots at the level of the shift become progressively stretched giving rise to bilateral sciatica and then neurological deficits.

The signs are at first confined to limited lumbar movement with local tenderness at the affected level on deep palpation. Later a step in the line of the spinous processes is palpable and then visible. In the worst forms a transverse fold of skin and excess soft tissue may develop. There may be symptoms of nerve root tension and then signs of nerve root deficit.

Lateral radiographs show the forward shift, but good quality oblique films will define the pathology between the superior and inferior facets of the neural arch. A lumbar myelogram will show any associated disc prolapse or nerve root compression. A CT or NMR scan may give additional information. In the stress fracture type of spondylolisthesis, the lesion in the neural arch may be invisible at first on oblique films. An isotopic bone scan may show a point of increased metabolic activity. 'Spondylolysis' is the term given to a neural arch with a stress fracture before any forward slip has occurred.

In the degenerative type treatment may be confined to a belt or a corset. In the stress fracture type a belt, corset or brace may allow the lesion to heal, although this is not a common result. If the lesion fails to heal or if symptoms worsen, an intertransverse spinal fusion is required. If there is a neurological deficit, a laminectomy is required as well.

Spinal fractures

At the time of injury every spinal fracture causes pain and limitation of movement. Fractures range from avulsion of the tip of a spinous process of a transverse process to a fracture dislocation of the column with displacement and paralysis. In nearly every case after the fracture has been reduced and has subsequently united, some chronic low back pain persists. There is scarring in the soft tissues and very often some residual malalignment of the fracture site and neighbouring joint surfaces.

The more general use of open reduction and internal fixation has improved results and has perhaps diminished the severity of post-traumatic backache, but it has not eliminated it.

Early treatment of minor stable spinal fractures is confined to temporary bed-rest, early regular physiotherapy and the support of a brace or belt until symptoms abate.

Early treatment of major and/or unstable fractures is usually by internal fixation from the posterior approach. Previously, spinal plates were applied to the spinous processes, but now Harrington rods hooked in to the lamina give better stability and durability. The treatment of fractures with paralysis has become a speciality on its own and involves surgery with a prolonged rehabilitation process.

After compression fractures of the vertebral bodies and fracture dislocations of the spinal column have occurred, degenerative changes in the nearby joints are usually radiographically visible within 1-2 years.

Patients with physically strenuous jobs require more time to return to work than those in sedentary occupations. Usually there is a significant and permanent diminution of the working capacity. Regular bursts of physiotherapy may keep the patient mobile and at work. A belt or a corset may be used for several months after the fracture has united.

Prolapsed intervertebral disc

A slipped disc (a prolapsed intervertebral disc, or a disc protrusion) is a herniation of the nucleus pulposus posteriorly or posterolaterally through the annulus fibrosus. This lesion occurs most often at the lumbosacral or lumbar 4/5 levels and in young adult life. However, any level of the spine can be affected and any age group. It is not as common as everyday conversation would suggest.

Lumbar flexion compresses the front of the disc and opens out the back of the disc. This tends to squeeze the nucleus pulposus posteriorly. High pressures are generated and are multiplied several times if a heavy object is lifted or carried.

Protrusion can occur by a sudden single violent

effort, but more usually it is a gradual process occurring from a multitude of smaller stresses, with a last final movement provoking a giving way of the annulus.

Posterolateral bulging of the disc may affect only a spinal nerve root, but midline bulging may affect one or more roots or the cauda equina nerve supply to the perineal organs. If the nucleus extrudes into the spinal canal to form a sequestrum, it can produce very sudden severe pain often with disturbance of bladder function or other neurological deficit.

After the prolapse has occurred, local inflammatory changes may increase the pressure surrounding the affected nerve root so that the least rise in intraspinal venous pressure will increase backache or sciatica, i.e. neck flexion, coughing, sneezing, laughing, defecation. The patient will complain of low back pain at first and sciatica shortly afterwards, but sometimes one or other of these components of pain is missing. Movement of the lumbar spine will also exacerbate the pain. The distribution of pain and/or the sensory and motor deficit below the knee will localise the nerve root, which is compressed by the disc prolapse. Above the knee it is not so diagnostic, as the dermatomes are so compressed in this part of the leg that much overlap occurs. Danger signals are bilateral sciatica, bladder dysfunction and more than one root involvement. To prevent permanent neurological loss, urgent surgical decompression is required.

Radiography is the chief means of investigation. Anteroposterior and lateral views of the disc space will show no changes in the early stages. Later the disc space will lose height and small osteophytes may be visible at the margins of the vertebral bodies. End plate sclerosis may eventually appear with osteoarthritic changes in the facet joints at the same level. Lumbar myelography will usually show posterior protrusions by compression of the column of contrast medium. Small protrusions may be shown only by compression of one or more nerve root pockets. Whole body computerised axial tomography (CT) and nuclear magnetic resonance imaging (NMRI) can now delineate precisely the relationship of disc, vertebrae, cauda equina and lateral root canals.

Central protrusion of disc material into the adjacent vertebral end plates is usually symptomless and is diagnosed on lateral films. This is termed a Schmorl's node.

With age and passage of time the nucleus becomes more dehydrated and fibrous, while the annulus heals with scar tissue. The volume of the prolapse is reduced and pain fades.

Conservative treatment aims to limit symptoms until the annulus heals and pain subsides. Trunk muscles are strengthened by isometric exercises. Angulation of the spine is diminished by attention to posture at work or in bed. Mechanical strains are lessened by losing any excessive weight and by avoiding lifting. External splinting by belts, corsets or casts may also limit spinal movement. Traction is of doubtful value and if applied in bed, merely helps to limit the patient's movement. Manipulation is also of very doubtful value in disc prolapses. To apply external force to a disc complex, the patient has to be caught unaware in a fully relaxed posture or must be anaesthetised. In either case, it is possible for the herniation of the nucleus to be enlarged by manipulation rather than diminished.

More active treatment may mean chemonucleolysis to shrink the nucleus, if the pathology is suitable. Otherwise the mainstay of surgical treatment has been discectomy by a posterior (laminectomy) approach. Later, symptoms from loss of disc height may arise because of root canal stenosis or localised instability of the disc complex. Such symptoms may be relieved by localised nerve root decompression +/− spinal fusion.

Spinal osteitis

Pyogenic spinal osteitis is rare and is often difficult to diagnose. It is frequently associated with diabetes, rheumatoid arthritis and immunosuppression. It may be iatrogenic from invasive investigations like discograms, etc. Like tuberculosis it regularly arises in the vertebral end plates from blood-stream spread, but it can occur in any part of the vertebral body. Very occasionally it can arise from contact with other infective foci in kidneys or lungs or from direct introduction from the exterior as in gunshot wounds, stabbing, etc.

The chief symptom is constant pain leading to limitation of movement. Signs can be obscure but local tenderness may be elicited by deep pressure or percussion. Root signs can be produced according to the site in the spinal column. Pus can track up and down the fascial planes forming a psoas abscess or bursting into the pleural cavity. A pyrexia may not be present and haematological changes of infection (i.e. raised ESR and WBC) are not always present either. Radiographs may show local rarefaction and diminution of a disc space. A bone isotope scan will show an increased uptake. A biopsy under image intensifiers may confirm the diagnosis and provide a profile of bacteriological sensitivity. If radiographs or a CT scan show little pus to be present, the appropriate antibiotic in large prolonged doses may suppress the infection. If pus or a sequestrum is present, surgery is required to evacuate the contents of the abscess.

Spinal tuberculosis

Tuberculous osteitis of the spine is usually secondary to tuberculous infection of the lungs or urinary tract. It is an insidious chronic infection of bone which leads to gradual destruction of the disc space and adjacent bone with the formation of caseous pus. A sharp kyphus will develop with long-term low-grade backache on a background of ill health. Caseous material will present in the neck from the cervical spine, but rarely presents from the thoracic spine unless it bursts into the lung or forms the rare empyema necessitas. From the lumbar spine pus tracks down the psoas major muscle and may form an abscess above or below the inguinal ligament.

In virulent infections and where a kyphus forms rapidly, paraplegia may gradually supervene ('Potts paraplegia'). This dangerous complication requires urgent treatment as soon as it is recognised.

Early radiographs show diminution of the disc space and local rarefaction of the end plates. Later there is loss of the disc space and local collapse of the adjacent vertebral bodies. If collapse continues, a sharp kyphus may form and calcified caseous material may lie anterolateral to the spinal column ('birds-nest' abscess in the thoracic spine or a psoas abscess in the lumbar region). A chest radiograph may show pulmonary tuberculosis and an intravenous pyelogram may show changes of tuberculosis in the renal tract. Treatment consists of rest and antibiotics. Surgery is limited to removal of pus, decompression of the spinal cord and internal splintage of skeletal defects.

Discitis

This term is given to a condition of acute severe low back pain associated with radiological evidence of calcification of a disc in the absence of infection. The condition is rare, but affects patients in youth or middle-age. The cause is unknown. There is a rapid onset of very severe low back pain without injury but aggravated by movement. There is no radiation of pain into the limbs, but any rise in spinal venous pressure such as caused by coughing, sneezing, straining, etc., can be agonising. There are no specific physical signs apart from the restriction of spinal movement and local tenderness on deep palpation. Very occasionally there may be a rapidly progressive paraplegia. Radiographs show variable calcification in the nucleus pulposus of usually only one disc, more often in the lower thoracic region than the lumbar region. If many discs are calcified, some other rare condition is present, such as fluorosis or alkaptonuria. There is no change in blood parameters, but every effort should be made to exclude pyogenic infection.

Treatment may require urgent decompression of the spinal cord and evacuation of the disc contents (like toothpaste). If the condition is less acute, bed-rest and analgesics may be all that is required for 1-2 weeks as the condition is usually self-limiting and long-term ill-effects are absent. Aspiration with or without the injection of an antibiotic or steroid under radiographic control is still unproven.

The acute discitis sometimes seen soon after disc surgery is likely to be caused by localised infection. There is severe pain on movement, often a pyrexia with a rise in the sedimentation rate and white blood count and on radiographs some loss of disc height, end plate sclerosis and no central calcification. The condition responds to antibiotics and bed-rest.

Pelvic sepsis

Pelvic sepsis is rarely a cause of chronic lower back ache felt in the pelvis, buttocks and perineum. The onset is often gradual and symptoms are present unremittingly day and night, whatever the posture. Coughing, sneezing, defecation and travel will all exacerbate the pain. There may be abnormalities of genitourinary or bowel function preceding the onset of backache. Women are more often affected than men and menstruation may worsen the symptoms. There is no sciatica and movements of the lumbar spine and hips are unrestricted.

Pelvic examination will elicit tenderness and swelling. Radiographs of the pelvis and lumbar spine are normal (unless there is some co-existing skeletal abnormality) but there may be other signs of infection, i.e. pyrexia, a raised ESR and a raised white-cell count. A vaginal or rectal discharge can be cultured. An ultrasound or CT scan of the pelvis may be diagnostic. Treatment lies with a gynaecologist or an abdominal surgeon.

Ankylosing spondylitis

Although the name suggests an infection, this is a chronic disease of unknown aetiology involving central cartilaginous and diarthrodial joints. It is not common but affects males at least eight times more commonly than females, beginning insidiously with low back pain and morning stiffness. Occasionally a shoulder or hip joint may be the first to be severely affected.

The early findings are limited movements in the lumbar and/or cervical regions and a diminished chest expansion. There may be other symptoms and signs indicating involvement of the eyes, large bowel, urethra, skin and nails.

Radiographs show sclerosis and then obliteration of the sacroiliac joints. The vertebral bodies appear squared off on the lateral views and later ossification occurs in the spinal ligaments. The costovertebral and manubiosternal joints fuse. The ESR is usually moderately raised but the rheumatoid factor is frequently absent. HLA-B27 antigen is present in 95 percent of patients.

Treatment is directed towards preventing fixed spinal flexion and towards maintaining chest expansion. Aspirin, naproxen and indomethacin are useful drugs for moderate pain control, but phenylbutzone is particularly effective. Unfortunately the latter carries the risk of agranulocytosis. Surgery is confined to synovectomy of a knee and replacement of the hip or knee, if these joints are severely affected. Patients whose spines have ankylosed in flexion may require a wedge osteotomy of the lumbar spine, to allow them to stand upright and to see ahead.

Aortic aneurysm

Aortic aneurysms can give rise to acute backache when they are enlarging, dissecting or leaking.

The most suspicious situation is the sudden onset of diffuse low back pain in an old man who may be at rest. He may have had symptoms or signs of vascular insufficiency before the onset of pain.

Signs in the peripheral vascular tree may be normal to begin with, but inequality of the pulses may be found with a unilateral or bilateral bruit over the femoral arteries. Femoral artery occlusion may follow quickly. The aneurysm may be palpable or elongated to form a midline pulsatile abdominal swelling and may be tender. A bruit may be present. The differential diagnosis is of an exacerbation of pre-existing lumbar spondylosis or a compression fracture of an osteoporotic spine, etc.

If an enlarging aneurysm is suspected, the patient should be admitted as an emergency case to the care of a vascular or abdominal surgeon.

Adenocarcinoma of the pancreas

This condition is rare, insidious, chronic and usually fatal if the presenting sign is backache. Other signs may be dyspepsia, malaise and loss of weight. The hormonal tumours of the pancreas do not present with backache and they produce many other symptoms and signs. The patient is usually middle-aged and complains of an upper lumbar midline ache that radiates around the abdomen. It is worsened when travelling and disturbs sleep. Often the patient will wake in the night to obtain relief by sitting up and hugging the knees. The chief differential diagnoses are lumbar spondylosis, aortic aneurysm and spinal metastases.

Diagnosis and treatment are beyond the scope of

this volume, but diffuse calcification is seen sometimes on the radiographs of the lumbar spine lying close to the anterior surfaces of L1 and L2.

Rectal carcinoma

Rectal carcinoma is a rare cause of low back pain felt in the sacrum and pelvis. If it has spread into the pelvis, there may be sciatica with a neurological deficit. The condition must be well advanced before skeletal symptoms appear and in virtually every case there are preceding bowel symptoms, i.e. alteration in bowel habit and the passage of mucus and/or blood.

A rectal examination is mandatory in every new patient with low back pain who has had some bowel or bladder disturbance. The walls of the rectum can be palpated and the shape, size and consistency of the prostate assessed. A rectal carcinoma may present as a broad-based polyp, a diffuse thickening of the rectal wall or an ulcer with thickened edges. In the latter case, blood is likely to be seen on the tip of the examining finger. Proctoscopy may enable internal haemorrhoids and/or a rectal ulcer to be visualised. Further investigation is best performed by a gastrointestinal surgeon rather than an orthopaedic surgeon.

It is possible for two pathologies to exist. The presence of a rectal or prostatic lesion should not delay routine investigation of other skeletal lesions higher in the lumbar spine.

Peptic ulceration

Peptic ulceration very rarely presents primarily as backache. Dyspepsia, heartburn, haematemesis or melaena are much more likely to draw attention to the underlying condition. However, chronic ulcers penetrating posteriorly in the duodenum may give rise to right-sided upper lumbar backache 1-2 hours after meals, often waking the patient at night.

There will be no abnormal signs on examining the spine but there may be upper midline tenderness in the abdomen. Endoscopy or a barium meal will identify the problem which may be solved by H_2 receptor blockers or surgery.

Renal lesions

Renal abnormalities may give rise to long-term unilateral backache felt in the loin and worsened by movement. There is no sciatica. The conditions are virtually all acquired, such as infections, hydronephrosis and tumours.

There may be a visible swelling or asymmetry in the

loin with some restriction of lumbar movements in all planes. There may be loin or abdominal tenderness and palpation may reveal an enlarged kidney. It is recognised by its shape, position and movement with respiration.

In this situation the renal lesion splints the lumbar spine but very rarely affects the skeleton otherwise. The exception is a perinephric abscess (tuberculosis or otherwise) which may give rise to local osteitis, or indeed may itself arise from a focus of vertebral osteitis.

If kidney disease is suspected, abdominal ultrasound and/or an intravenous pyelogram will give confirmation but there may be co-existing skeletal abnormalities in the lumbar spine (i.e. degenerative changes) which may or may not contribute to symptoms and signs. If kidney disease is confirmed, then treatment is directed first to this condition and later to the spine.

Lumbar spondylosis

Lumbar spondylosis encompasses the degenerative changes that come with age and which are accelerated by deformity, asymmetry, injury and chronic disease. They consist of loss of disc height and dehydration of the nucleus pulposus with osteophyte formation at the attachments of the annulus fibrosus. In the posterior joints there is loss of articular cartilage and local osteophyte formation which can compress the local nerve root canal causing pain and/or neurological deficit. These osteophytes and those on the posterior margin of the disc can combine with slight buckling of the ligamentum flavum to produce stenosis of the lumbar vertebral canal.

Lumbar spondylosis in radiographs is seen first at the thoracolumbar levels in men of 30-40 years of age who have hard physical jobs. In these cases it spreads downwards to affect all levels of the lumbar spine; otherwise degenerative changes arise at localised sites of injury or disc herniation. There is pain and stiffness on movement from rest and sometimes localised sciatica. Occasionally it is difficult to differentiate the causes of sciatic pain in the second half of life, especially claudication, which can be ischaemic or neurogenic in origin (*see* lumbar stenosis).

Treatment consists of weight reduction, analgesics and physiotherapy. Severe pain on movement may be relieved by the temporary use of a corset or belt. If severe, prolonged sciatica can be localised accurately to one or two root canals, these may be decompressed by surgical removal of osteophytes. Neurogenic claudication can be relieved by a multilevel laminectomy. Unisegmental lumbar spondylosis may be temporarily relieved by localised spinal fusion, but

adjoining levels soon become painful and the final state may be as bad as the first.

Lumbar stenosis

Lumbar stenosis is defined as constriction of the spinal canal in the lumbar region from congenital or acquired causes. It is not common. There is a wide variation in the capacity of the spinal canal in patients who are otherwise normal clinically and radiologically, but those with smaller spinal canals are more likely to have symptoms which result from nerve root compression. These changes can result from Down's syndrome, osteogenesis imperfecta, acromegaly, fractures and, most commonly, lumbar spondylosis.

The symptoms are low back pain with unilateral or bilateral sciatica worsened by exercise and relieved by rest (spinal claudication). If present when walking, it is relieved by sitting down or bending forwards. This feature with the presence of peripheral pulses will differentiate it from ischaemic claudication, in which the peripheral pulses are absent and which is relieved merely by resting.

The advent of CT and NMR scans has revolutionised the diagnosis and surgical treatment of lumbar stenosis. With these tools the exact configuration of the spinal canal and the emergent root canals can be shown on screen and films. Previously, measurements from conventional films and inspection of myelographic films gave uncertain information. The aim of surgery is to enlarge the spinal canal and decompress the cauda equina by laminectomy. At the same time any osteophytes identified as compressing laterally emergent nerve root(s) are removed.

Primary spinal bone tumours

These are rarities. Secondary tumours are far more common. Of the benign primary tumours, osteoid osteomata and osteoblastomata usually arise in the neural arches or transverse processes and are difficult to diagnose, because radiographic changes are slow to develop in the young patient who complains of long-term intermittent backache. Osteomata or osteochondromata do not cause pain until they impinge on adjacent structures. Similar tumours may be present in other parts of the appendicular skeleton. They occur before 30 years of age. Osteoclastomata, haemangiomata and aneurysmal bone cysts have been reported in the spine and are on the borderline of malignancy. They usually present with backache and are visible on the initial radiographs.

Primary malignant spinal bone tumours are as rare as benign tumours but may be a chondrosarcoma or an osteosarcoma. Again backache is the chief presenting symptom and stiffness the chief presenting sign. Rarely there may be localised deformity or tenderness and signs of distal neurological deficit. Tumours of the spinal column are investigated chiefly by radiographic techniques i.e. myelography, tomography, CT scans and NMR scans. A bone isotopic scan is useful to prove the increased local uptake of isotope and the absence of other areas of increased uptake. A tissue biopsy is vital for planning treatment. Usually a closed biopsy under image intensifiers will provide sufficient material for histological diagnosis. When all available evidence is gathered, definitive treatment can be planned with an oncologist, a surgeon and a radiotherapist (or other specialists depending on the individual circumstances of the patient).

Primary intraspinal tumours are rare and nearly all are benign i.e. neurofibromata, ependymomata, dermoids, etc. They give rise to back pain on movement and at night. Eventually, a neurological deficit will appear. If this is a bladder paralysis, an urgent laminectomy is needed.

Secondary bone tumours: spinal metastases

Secondary bone tumours or spinal metastases are by far the most common spinal neoplasms and mostly occur in the second half of life. Usually the primary site is well known to the patient and medical staff but sometimes the secondary spinal deposit is the presenting feature of the primary pathology. Metastases are mostly from the breast, lung and prostate, in that order of frequency. However, tumours of the kidney and thyroid can produce spinal secondaries. More rarely, tumours of the gastrointestinal tract and bladder can metastasise to the spine. All these, except the prostatic metastases, are osteolytic and can lead rapidly to a pathological fracture and vertebral collapse. Spinal cord compression is a frequent complication with the rapid onset of paraplegia.

Pain is the first and major feature; often of very sudden onset. The patient may look ill, pale and tired or even cachectic. A small tender kyphus is often present and there may be some neurological deficit below the lesion. Movements of the lumbar spine are restricted or absent. If a secondary metastasis is suspected, the primary site should be sought at the first physical examination. This includes a rectal and/or a vaginal examination.

The single most useful investigation is a bone isotope scan but conventional radiography is usually performed first. This may show loss of bone outlines (including loss of a pedicle) with compression of the vertebral body, if 50 per cent or more of local bone is lost. Local soft-tissue swelling with generalised osteoporosis may indicate myelomatosis, but the osteoporosis alone may be merely an indicator of age or inactivity. A bone isotope scan is usually performed immediately afterwards on the suspicion of metastases, as it will be positive some time before changes are seen on conventional radiographic films.

Localised osteosclerosis is usually a sign of a prostatic metastasis. Blood is taken for a biochemical screen, including prostate specific antigen erythrocyte. Hypercalcaemia may be dangerous and require urgent treatment. A raised sedimentation rate and serum protein level suggests myelomatosis.

If there are signs of spinal cord compression, urgent decompressive laminectomy is required +/− internal fixation +/− bone grafting to stabilise the spinal column. This will allow histological diagnosis from biopsy specimens.

If there is no sign of incipient paraplegia, other investigations can be conducted, i.e. isotopic bone scan, CT scan. When a full range of information is available, treatment can be planned with surgical, radiotherapeutic, oncological and radiological colleagues.

Myelomatosis

This condition is caused by a proliferation of plasma cells of the marrow and usually affects the axial skeleton and the proximal limb segments in the second half of life. The cause is not known. It is presumed that the condition has been present for some years before it becomes clinically evident. The structural defects of myelomatosis result from expansion of the tumour in the marrow and the steady erosion of cortical bone. Usually many vertebral bodies are affected and are liable to compression fractures from trivial stresses. Extra dural growth of the tumour and involvement of the neural arches may lead to the rapid onset of paraplegia when a vertebral body collapses.

The patient, often elderly and if a woman, often osteoporotic, may complain of an increase of longstanding backache. There may be irregular skeletal pains and an increasing kyphosis with loss of height. Sometimes a minor injury can cause agonising backache and the rapid onset of numbness and weakness in the legs. Occasionally, a pathological fracture of the humerus or femur may precede vertebral compression fractures.

Radiographs show localised irregular osteoporosis with erosion of cortical bone surfaces from within. There may be compression of one or more vertebral bodies. Osteolytic lesions may be present also in the limb girdles and proximal limb bones. The lesions in the skull have a characteristic punched out appearance.

There is accompanying anaemia and hypergamma-globulinaemia. The uniquely abnormal protein produced by the tumour may leak into the urine (Bence-Jones protein). The erythrocyte sedimentation rate is greatly raised and abnormal plasma cells may be present in the circulation. If there is much bone destruction, hypercalcaemia may be present.

The treatment of a pathological fracture with spinal cord compression is by urgent decompression by a wide laminectomy. Internal fixation, if possible, may be a useful option at this time. The very major thoracoabdominal approaches with bone grafting and internal fixation operations for lumbar and thoracic fractures are still experimental.

If the diagnosis of myelomatosis is made before a fracture occurs, local radiotherapy and systemic chemotherapy are required, together with the external support of a brace or corset.

Despite intensive treatment the condition is always fatal within 1-2 years.

Osteoporosis

Osteoporosis is defined as the gradual loss of bone with both the calcium and protein components being deficient. This is in contrast to osteomalacia which is a loss of calcium from normal bone matrix. Osteoporosis occurs naturally after the menopause in women and about 10 years later in men. It can also occur from inactivity due to prolonged splintage, paralysis, arthritis or simple lack of exercise. It has been found to occur in astronauts living for long periods in zero gravity. If osteoporosis is severe, pathological fractures may occur. These are most often seen in the vertebral bodies, in the neck of the femur and at the lower end of the radius. Paralysed or arthritic limbs are easily broken by trivial violence, if the skeleton is osteoporotic.

The diagnosis of osteoporosis can be made on conventional radiographs when about 50 per cent of normal bone density is lost. Comparisons by radiography are virtually impossible because of so many variables. As a research tool photo absorption spectrometry of the lower radius is more reliable. Pathological fractures are likely to occur when 70 per cent of normal adult density is lost.

The osteoporotic spine gives rise to low-grade chronic backache with increasing long-segment kyphosis and loss of height. It is usually most obvious in the thoracic region, so that the patient develops a position of flexion (dowager's hump). In the lumbar region the loss of height causes the 11th and 12th ribs to impinge on the pelvis and leads to a protuberant abdomen and redundant folds of skin. Vertebral compression fractures can occur spontaneously or from trivial violence. Severe pain is present, but a spinal paralysis is very rare. Pain gradually resolves over several weeks.

Pathological fractures will heal satisfactorily and in average time, but usually with persistent deformity. Maintenance of reduction is extremely difficult because of the local fragility and compression of trabeculae around the fracture. Internal fixation, with or without bone grafting, is often difficult or hazardous. Malunion is often an acceptable alternative in the very elderly.

The onset of osteoporosis of old age can be postponed by vigorous activity if the heart, lungs and joints allow. There is debate about the value of oestrogen replacement therapy in post-menopausal women. Small daily doses of oestrogen may delay the onset and can halt the process if given after the onset, but reversal is uncertain. There seems to be a small increase in endometrial carcinoma as a result of long-term oestrogen therapy. If the diet is deficient in calcium, protein and vitamin D, then supplements may delay the progression of osteoporosis.

Osteomalacia

Osteomalacia is defined as the loss of calcification in the adult skeleton caused by lack of vitamin D. It occurs in those on diets deficient in vitamin D or in those whose skin is shielded from sunlight. It can also occur in those with malabsorption syndromes or with genetic renal tubular defects. The childhood equivalent is rickets.

Osteomalacic bones become soft and elastic and will bend under gravity. This gives rise to a kyphus, deformed pelves, coxa vara and bowed legs. There may be a spontaneous onset of pain to accompany the deformities. Bands of decalcification occur in any part of the skeleton but are most often seen around the shoulder and pelvic girdles. These are often termed 'pseudo-fractures' or 'Looser's zones'. On radiographs osteomalacia can be diagnosed by the characteristic deformities, the pseudo-fractures and fish-tailed vertebrae. There is often a generalised loss of bone density. The serum calcium levels are depressed, while the phosphate and alkaline phosphatase levels are elevated.

The disease can be arrested or cured by giving vitamin D orally in most cases. Those with malabsorption or renal tubular disorders may require vitamin D in large doses, i.e. 1.25mg daily, although overdosage can lead to renal failure. Surgery is not necessary, except to strengthen bowed legs after the biochemical abnormality has been corrected.

Psychological aspects of back pain

Physiologically, pain is a warning system of bodily dysfunction, but on the psychological level it can be a cry for sympathy or an expression of guilt. At a deeper level aggression may be sublimated to pain.

The back is known to be an area in which physicians have difficulty in providing relief and is part of the body which is never seen and is difficult to touch. It is turned for defence, used for punishment and enclosed in love or sympathy.

The premorbid personality may lead to the back pain being seen as a confirmation of lack of self-esteem. Deformity may be seen as a punishment for a sin and is often culturally influenced. Indeed the family may reinforce this perception. Physical illness and disability may satisfy security and dependence needs without stigmatising the patient, because the sick role is accepted by most societies. In addition, the patient may wish to continue the financial support which the disability allows, either through insurance, the government or the family.

Patients whose pain is mostly psychological have difficulty in reaching any relationship of trust or confidence in their physician. They often appear to have an attitude of suspicion and may blame another person for their troubles. Their history is often vague with bizarre or emotional descriptions. They may present an expression, posture, or voice of depression. They may show inappropriate effects such as complaining of severe pain without appearing to be in pain. They are easily distracted to symptoms in other systems and may boast of their terrible pain and its effects. The physical examination may provoke histrionic displays, a worsening of signs on formal examination, and an unanatomical distribution of pain. A pyschiatric evaluation may help to unravel symptoms and signs in such patients, while psychiatric treatment may relieve some features.

History taking

'The patient will tell you the diagnosis if you are prepared to listen'—an aphorism nearly a century old; but no amount of talking and listening will localise a specific painful spinal joint. The age, sex and occupation of the patient will immediately exclude certain conditions; an old woman will not have carcinoma of the prostate but is more likely to be osteoporotic. A young man is more likely to have ankylosing spondylitis than a young woman. A young person performing strenuous tasks is more likely to have a disc prolapse than a secondary tumour. With experience the history is tailored to the first clues offered by the patient.

Most orthopaedic histories are very brief and encompass all the necessary information—'I broke my shin this afternoon when I was kicked during a football match. I have never been in hospital before'. However, they become longer as the patient grows older. The gradual onset of musculoskeletal pain in the trunk or limbs always requires a detailed history of the function of the main bodily systems and past medical history. Most orthopaedic surgeons concentrate on the following salient points:

- Duration of pain
- Laterality or localisation
- Exacerbating factors
- Presence of leg pain
- Function of the bladder
- Any other bodily disturbance
- Previous injury or illness
- Effect of any previous treatment

In patients with a long history of low back pain, previous investigation and treatment must be recorded together with the effects of such treatment.

A questionnaire can be time saving, if completed *before* the consultation.

An example of a questionnaire appears below.

Name: _____ Unit No _____

DISABILITY INDEX QUESTIONNAIRE

When your back or your leg hurts, you may find it difficult and painful to do some of the things you normally do.

This questionnaire contains some sentences that people have used to describe themselves when they have back pain or leg pain. When you read them, you may find that some stand out because they describe you today. As you read the questionnaire, think of yourself today. When you read a sentence that describes you today, put a tick against it. If the sentence does not describe you, then leave the space blank and go on to the next one.

Remember, only tick the sentence if you are sure that it describes you today.

I stay at home most of the time because of my back pain/leg pain

I change position frequently to try and get my back/leg comfortable

I walk more slowly than usual because of my back pain/leg pain

Because of my back pain/leg pain, I am not doing any of the jobs I usually do around the house

Because of my back pain/leg pain, I use a handrail to climb up stairs

Because of my back pain/leg pain, I lie down to rest more often

Because of my back pain/leg pain, I have to hold on to something to get out of easy chair

Because of my back pain/leg pain, I try to get other people to do things for me

I get dressed more slowly than usual, because of my back pain/leg pain

I only stand up for short periods of time, because of my back pain/leg pain

Because of my back pain/leg pain, I try not to bend or kneel down

I find it difficult to get out of a chair, because of my back pain/leg pain

My back/leg is painful almost all the time

I find it difficult to turn over in bed, because of my back pain/leg pain

My appetite is not very good, because of my back pain/leg pain

I have trouble putting on my socks (or stockings), because of the pain in my back/leg

I only walk short distances, because of my back pain/leg pain

I sleep less well, because of my back pain/leg pain

Because of my back pain/leg pain, I get dressed with help from someone else

I sit down for most of the day, because of my back pain/leg pain

I avoid heavy jobs around the house, because of my back pain/leg pain

Because of my back pain/leg pain, I am more irritable and bad tempered with people than usual

Because of my back pain/leg pain, I climb up stairs more slowly than usual

I stay in bed most of the time, because of my back pain/leg pain

My back/leg pain increases, if I sit on the toilet

My back/leg pain increases, if I cough or sneeze

PAIN RATING SCALE

Now we want you to give us an idea of just how bad your pain is at the moment.

We want you to put a tick by the words that describe your pain best.

Remember, we want to know how bad your pain is at the moment.

The pain is almost unbearable.

Very bad pain.

Quite bad pain.

Moderate pain.

Little pain.

No pain at all.

Thank you for answering the questionnaire.

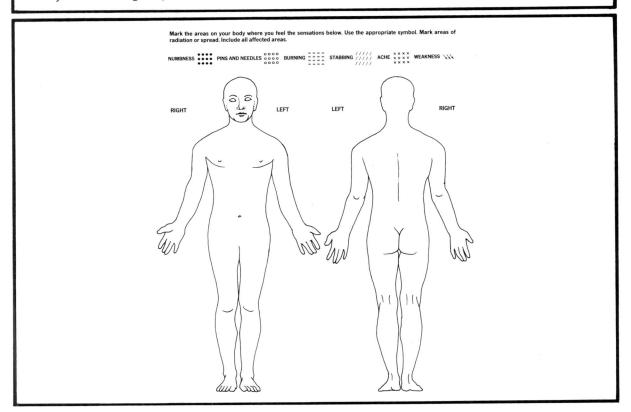

Mark the areas on your body where you feel the sensations below. Use the appropriate symbol. Mark areas of radiation or spread. Include all affected areas.

NUMBNESS   PINS AND NEEDLES   BURNING   STABBING   ACHE   WEAKNESS

RIGHT   LEFT   LEFT   RIGHT

Physical examination

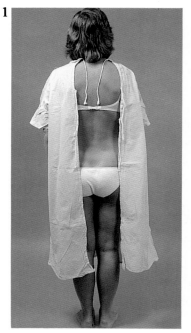

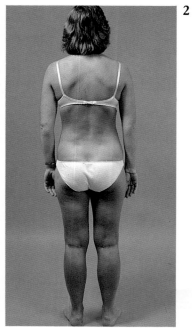

1 The patient should be standing and stripped down to underclothes. Women may prefer to use a surgical gown.

2 If the gown is removed, asymmetry of the shoulders or legs may be seen more easily from the back view.

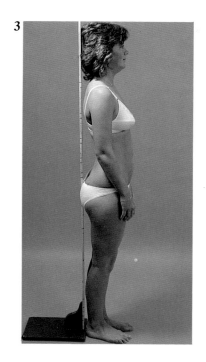

3 Side view will show any hollow (lordosis) or any flexion (kyphosis) of the spine.

4 Later pregnancy will induce a compensatory lumbar lordosis particularly in taller, thinner women. This may be a source of back ache relieved very rapidly by delivery.

A short segment lordosis may be caused by a spondylolisthesis. Viewed from the back, a ridge of soft tissue may be visible at the lower edge of the lordosis.

A long segment lumbar lordosis is usually caused by obesity or by fixed flexion deformities of the hips.

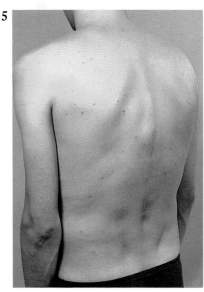

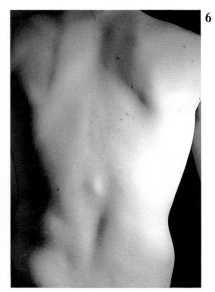

5 Young man with a kyphus and a scar from internal fixation of a fracture.

6 A sharp kyphus is indicative of localised disease, i.e. trauma, infection or tumour.

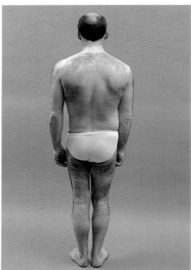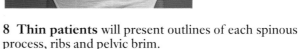

7 Tension on the roots of the sciatic nerve may cause the patient to tilt his spine to one side to relieve the pain. This man has a lumbosacral disc lesion.

A short leg which is not balanced by a shoe raise will cause a spinal tilt, which if not relieved over a long period will cause secondary low back pain.

8 Thin patients will present outlines of each spinous process, ribs and pelvic brim.

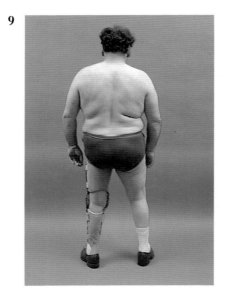

9 The skeletal contours of obese patients will be obscured, but nearly all will have a lumbar lordosis to balance the weight of the abdomen. This man has an artificial left leg.

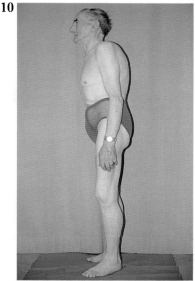

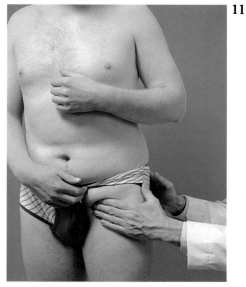

10 Long-segment smooth kyphoses in old age are usually seen in the upper thoracic spine of old women (dowager's hump). This old man has a similar deformity caused by gradual vertebral body compression from osteoporosis. A smooth kyphus in a young person is usually caused by thoracic vertebral epiphysitis (Scheuermann's disease). This is most commonly seen in tall males with tight hamstrings. The condition is rarely painful.

11 The hernial orifices are best examined with the patient standing and the underclothes removed. The genitalia may also require to be examined. A complaint of pain in the groin may result from a variety of causes.

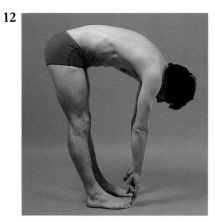

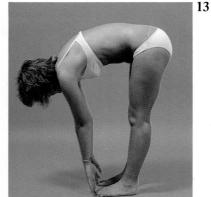

12 Side view of a patient bending forwards. In a normal lumbar spine forward flexion will result in a smooth lumbar curvature involving all the segments. Whether the patient can touch his/her toes depends more on the relative lengths of legs and arms and the laxity of the hamstring muscles than lumbar spinal flexion.

13 Measurement of movements of lumbar flexion are prone to wide variations of observer error. The distance between the fingertips and the floor depends on several factors, apart from the degree of lumbar flexion. The increasing length between L1 spinous process and the lower sacrum is a better measurement, but is difficult to reproduce exactly on two or more examinations separated by days or weeks. This girl bends forward by flexing her hips and not by flexing her lumbar spine. This is a variation of normal.

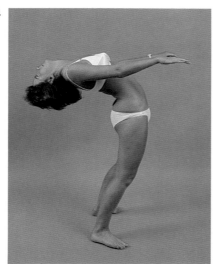

14 Extension of the lumbar spine is variable. Hypermobile people can become gymnasts or dancers. Most young people can arch their backs, but those with a fixed lumbar lordosis from obesity or fixed flexion of the hips cannot extend at all from their normal posture, which is already a position of maximum extension.

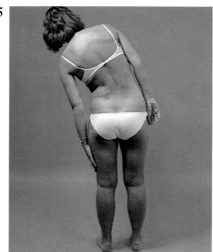

15 Lateral flexion of the spine should be performed without any element of forward flexion. In the presence of nerve root damage or tension, lateral flexion towards the side of the lesion is usually normal but away from the side of the lesion, is usually restricted and painful.

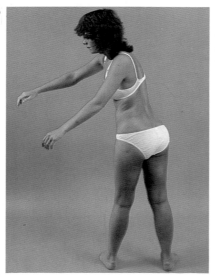

16 Rotation of the lumbar spine is often unrestricted when flexion and/or extension is painful. Rotation alone may cause pain if the patient has an injury, infection or neoplasm.

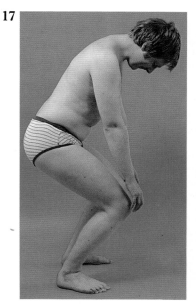

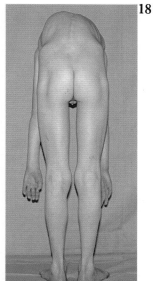

17 This patient has a lumbar disc lesion and his lumbar spine is held involuntarily in a straight position by reflex contraction of the spinal extensors. This relieves pain from the abnormal disc. He bends by hip flexion.

In rising from a bent position the patient bends his knees to allow hip extension, before using his spinal extensors to complete the act of becoming vertical (reversed spinal rhythm).

18 A boy with a scoliotic spine bending forwards. The secondary asymmetry of the ribs is visible and accentuated by flexion.

Scoliosis can be congenital or acquired, but in early adolescence it often has no discernible cause. In girls it can appear suddenly and rapidly progress to an obvious deformity.

An idiopathic scoliosis is usually painless until after the third decade.

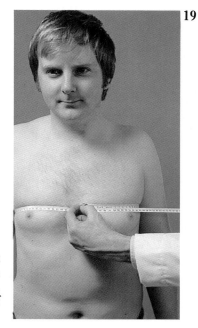

19 Chest expansion is measured before the patient lies down. This is important in young men with diffuse low back pain and morning stiffness. A loss of chest expansion may be an additional sign of ankylosing spondylitis.

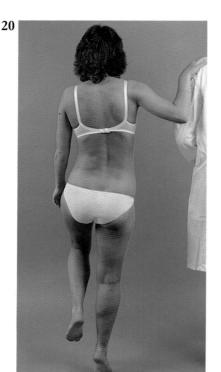

20 The power of the calf musculature can be tested while the patient is standing. Usually this muscle group is so strong that it cannot be tested by the examiner in any other way. The patient steadies herself with one hand and is asked to stand on tiptoe on one foot. She is then asked to lower and lift the heel, rising and falling in quick succession. The average person can perform a sequence of 10 lifts without difficulty. This is reduced if the muscles are weak (S1 root supply). The other leg is then tested.

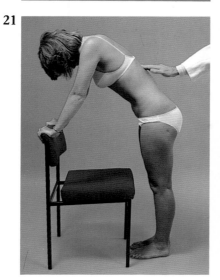

21 Palpitation of the spine is usually easier with the patient bending forward and holding the back of the chair, than if she is standing up. This posture opens out the interspinous spaces and does not allow the patient to move forward so easily in response to the examiner's touch. Individual spinous processes can be felt and soft tissue tenderness well localised.

22 Ankle reflexes (Achilles tendon reflex S1) can be elicited with the patient kneeling, but relaxation can be improved by the patient positioning the knees on the rear of the seat and holding the back of the chair by the hands. This is an easy way to compare the ankle reflexes. An alternative way of obtaining these reflexes is with the patient supine (vide infra). (See Figs. 54 and 55.)

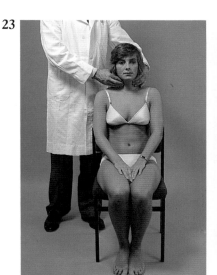

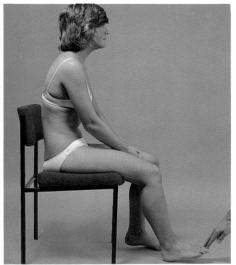

23 A rise in spinal venous pressure may irritate a nerve root and give rise to pain in the leg, with a distribution such as to allow localisation in the spine. This may occur in coughing or defecation but can be elicited by gentle jugular venous compression. The patient must be reassured and gentle pressure applied by the fingertips over the carotid sheaths. The carotid arteries must not be occluded, because the patient may become unconscious and even death may occur.

24 The strength of the extensors of the toes can be tested if the patient extends the knee and rests the heel on the ground. The examiner can attempt to plantar flex the foot against the patient's resistance.

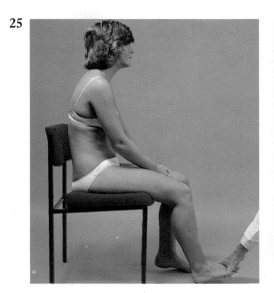

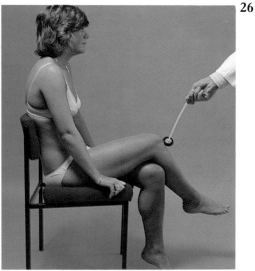

25 The same tests can be applied to the dorsiflexors of the ankle.

26 The knee reflex (L3/4) can be elicited by having the patient sitting with the knees crossed. This posture stretches the quadriceps, but sometimes the patient must be distracted before she can relax sufficiently. Left and right reflexes can be compared but there are other ways of eliciting this reflex with the patient supine (vide infra). (See Figs. 52 and 53.)

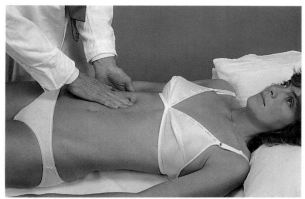

27 **The liver edge** is frequently palpable in children or adults, but enlargement of greater than 1-2 cm below the costal margin is abnormal. The features of the enlargement should be noted, i.e. tenderness, irregularity, etc. The examining fingers are pressed gently below the margin of the ribs and the movement of the liver edge with respiration is sought. A grossly enlarged liver may be overlooked if the free edge is many centimetres below the costal margin.

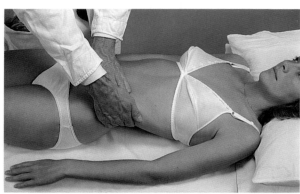

28 **The kidney** is sought by placing one hand in the loin and gently lifting the tissues forward to the palpating hand held gently on the abdominal wall. An enlarged kidney may be felt to move on respiration.

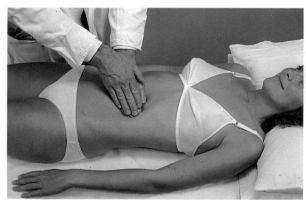

29 **The spleen** is normally hidden under the left costal margin and moves downwards on respiration. It may be palpated by fingertips pressed lightly under the costal cartilages. The edge of a very large spleen may be many centimetres below the costal margin.

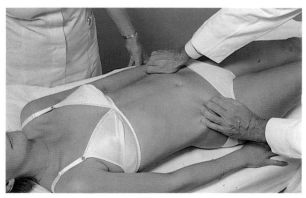

30 **Compression of the sacroiliac joint.** This joint can be stressed in a number of ways. By holding the anterior superior iliac spines, the examiner can compress or distract the pelvis. This may produce pain in an injured or infected sacroiliac joint.

31 Distractions of the sacroiliac joint. This joint is one of the strongest in the human body and nowadays is only very infrequently the source of low back pain. Pain is often referred to the posterior aspect of the joint and the spinal extensor origins may be tender. A sacroiliac strain probably does not exist except after very major trauma, when there are fractures of the anterior part of the pelvis.

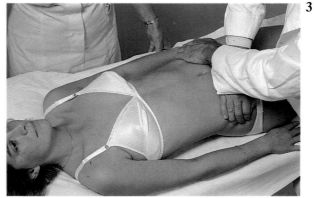

32 The sacroiliac joints can be tested by asking the patient to clasp one knee with the hip flexed. The other leg is extended at the hip over the end of the couch (Gaenslen's test). Pain around the sacroiliac region is diagnostic of local pathology such as injury, infection or trauma (see **61**).

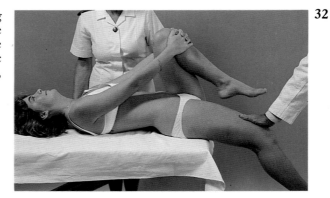

33 If the sciatic nerve roots are under severe tension, merely lifting the head off the couch may cause low back pain or pain in the leg.

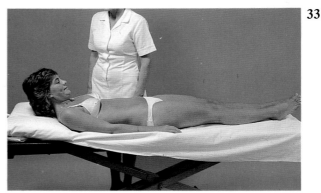

34 Occasionally, sciatica and claudication can be confused, particularly if the claudication is neurogenic rather than ischaemic. It is important to palpate the peripheral pulses in all patients.

The dorsalis pedis pulse is usually felt between the bases of the 1st and 2nd metatarsals but the anatomy is not always constant; the artery may be palpable anywhere over the dorsum of the foot. Nevertheless, in cases of difficulty, the termination of the anterior tibial artery is constantly present anterior to the ankle and lateral to the tibialis anterior tendon.

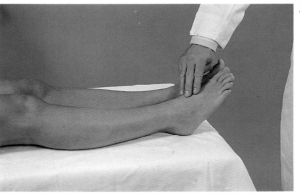

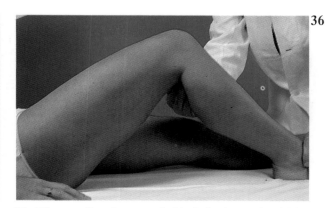

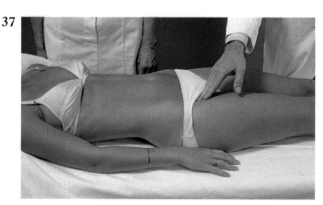

35 If a dorsalis pedis pulse is impalpable, the presence of the posterior tibial pulse posterior to the medial malleolus should be sought.

36 The popliteal artery behind the knee should be palpated, if no pulses are palpable at the foot or if there are other signs of ischaemia (i.e. pallor on elevation, lividity on dependency, loss of hair, etc.).

The knee should be flexed to an angle of 90 degrees and relaxed. The examining fingertip should be directed towards the tibial tuberosity.

37 If no pulse is palpable behind the knee, it should be sought in the femoral artery in the groin at the midpoint of the inguinal ligament. The quality of pulsation of the femoral arteries can be compared in each groin.

If there is doubt about the blood supply of the legs, both groins should be auscultated. The presence of a bruit indicates a disturbance of blood flow often resulting from atheroma. In a young person absent leg pulses with normal arm pulses usually means coarctation of the aorta.

On palpation of the abdomen it is sometimes difficult to differentiate between transmitted pulsation and expansile pulsation. A thin patient with a lumbar lordosis may have a normal aorta which is very easily palpable. Any palpable aorta more than 4 cm in width is certainly pathological (usually atheromatous). If it is enlarged and tender, it may be leaking or infected. In such instances the advice of a vascular surgeon is required urgently.

38 Hip posture and movements. This illustration demonstrates a test for hip rotation in flexion. Fixed flexion of the hip(s) may lead to a secondary lumbar lordosis to allow the patient to stand vertical. After a time the lordosis can become fixed and painful. Indeed some lumbar spines are fixed permanently in maximum extension.

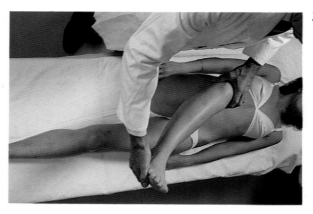

Fixed flexion of the hip is tested by asking the patient to bend both hips with the knees over the abdomen. One hand of the examiner is passed under the lumbar spine to ensure it is flattened onto the couch. The other hand of the examiner holds the knee on the side not to be tested. The patient is then asked to straighten out the free leg (that to be tested). If he can bring it flat on the couch, there is no fixed flexion. If he cannot, the degree of fixed flexion can be estimated by eye or measured by a goniometer (Thomas's test).

Adduction of the hips is tested by asking the patient to cross one leg over the other, while the examiner holds the pelvis to prevent it tilting sideways. Adduction in the supine position always involves some flexion as well (unless the patient has lost one leg). There is a normal range of 20-30 degrees.

Abduction of the hip is tested in a similar manner; the examiner holding the opposite side of the pelvis to detect the point when it tilts at the limit of abduction. Children are more mobile than adults.

Rotation of the hip can also be tested with the hips and knees flexed. In this posture with the knees together outward (lateral) movement of the foot shows internal rotation of the hip. Conversely inward (medial) movement of the foot shows external rotation of the hip. Hip rotation slowly deteriorates throughout life, although patients who continue to sit in the W position until they are adults retain an excess range of internal rotation.

Pain in the buttock, thigh or groin may arise from abnormalities in the hip; for this reason the range of motion of the hip joints should be tested. One hip is compared with the other. Flexion is usually possible beyond a right angle, provided the knee is flexed as well. Young people can kiss their knees.

39 Straight leg raising (SLR) is a test for tension on the sciatic nerve roots. The patient is asked to relax and, with the knee straight, the heel is lifted by the examiner until pain is felt. The site of the pain is important, so the patient is asked to say where the pain is worst. If pain is in the back or buttock, a central disc prolapse may be the cause. If the pain is felt at the back of the thigh, the only abnormality may be tight hamstrings; this can be tested by the bow-string manoeuvre (vide infra). If the pain is felt below the knee, it may correspond to the lumbosacral dermatomes; this forms an important localising sign. Sometimes pain is produced in the opposite leg as well and this is an indication of pathology within the spinal canal.

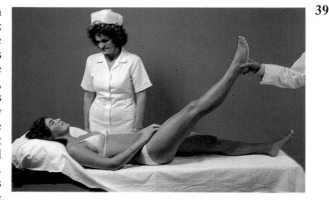

In the absence of spinal or hip pathology, SLR may be carried to the vertical position. In patients with long hamstrings or joint hypermobility, SLR may exceed an angle of 90 degrees.

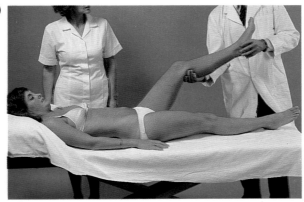

40 The bow-string test is performed by flexing the hip to 45-60 degrees with the knee flexed. Passive extension of the knee may then reproduce pain in the affected branches of the sciatic nerve.

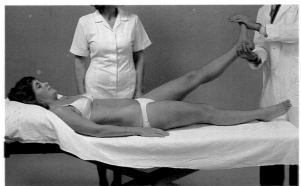

41 Lasegue's test. The sciatic nerve normally stretches 2-3 cm when lifting the leg from the horizontal to the vertical position. Pathology in or near the spine may prevent this by causing pain. True sciatic tension can be confirmed by lifting the leg to the point just below pain. Passive dorsiflexion of the foot may then reproduce pain by stretching the sciatic nerve just a fraction more (Lasegue's test). The localisation of pain below the knee is particularly significant.

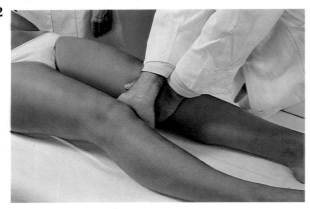

42 The power of hip adduction (L2 3 roots) can be tested by asking the patient to squeeze her knees together against the resistance of the examiner's hand.

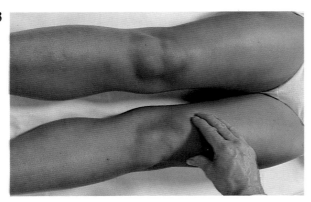

43 The relative bulk and firmness of the quadriceps can be tested by palpating the lower part of the thigh as the patient extends the knee as strongly as she can.

44 The strength of the quadriceps (L3 4 roots) can be crudely tested by asking the patient to keep the knee straight, while the examiner tries to bend the knee over the fulcrum of his forearm.

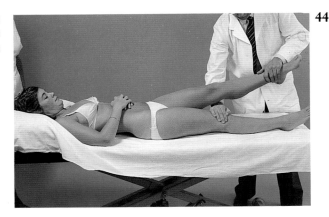

45 The power of the big toe extensors (L5 root) can be tested by asking the patient to draw up the toes against the examiner's resistance.

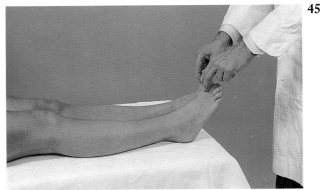

46 The power of eversion of the foot (peroneal muscles, L5 S1 roots) is tested by asking the patient to push the outer border of the foot against the examiner's hand.

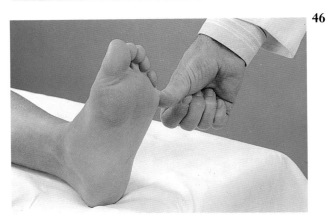

47 The power of inversion of the foot (L4 5 roots) can be tested by asking the patient to push the inner border of the foot inwards against the resistance of the examiner's hand.

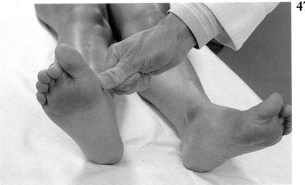

33

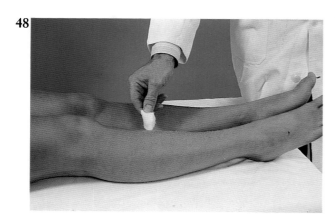

48 Sensation in the legs should be tested by light touch, fine touch (pin-prick) pain and proprioception. The dermatomes overlap considerably and the examiner's findings are totally dependent on the patient's co-operation. The perception of light touch is accentuated by the presence of hairs and thin skin. Thick hairless skin on the sole of the foot is often less sensitive.

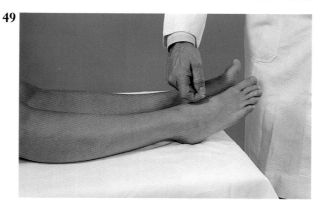

49 Pin-prick sensation is also accentuated by the presence of hairs and the absence of thick layers of keratin. It is also dependent upon the pressure with which the pin-point is applied and a spring-loaded pin will give a more constant stimulus.

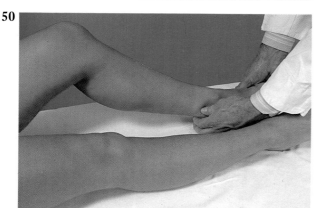

50 Sensations of pain can be provoked by pinching a skin fold or squeezing the Achilles tendon. These actions cause no permanent damage to the patient and pain is relieved immediately by relaxing the pressure.

Posterior column sensations of heat, cold and joint proprioception are not often tested in the legs when the patient's complaint is backache. Nevertheless, they are appropriate in some situations, e.g. Tabes dorsalis or Charcot's spine.

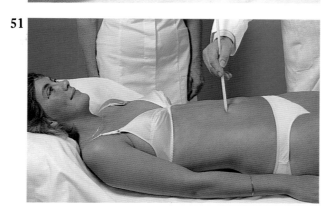

51 The abdominal musculature will reflexly contract if a pointed object is drawn up the abdomen. The reflex can be elicited from both sides of the abdominal wall. Absence of the reflex indicates pathology in the lower thoracic segments of the spinal cord.

52 The knee reflexes can be elicited in the supine position, if the patient can relax and give the whole weight of her legs into the examiner's forearm behind the knee (L3 4 roots).

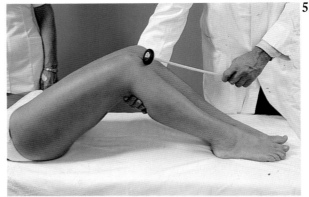

53 If relaxation is not possible at first, the patient's attention can be distracted by asking her to link her hands across her chest and try to pull them apart. This usually produces relaxation of the quadriceps.

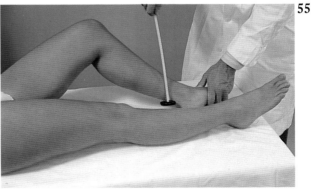

54 The ankle reflex can be elicited by the examiner dorsiflexing the patient's foot and striking the back of his hand with the tendon hammer (L5 S1 roots). The patient's ankle extensors should be relaxed.

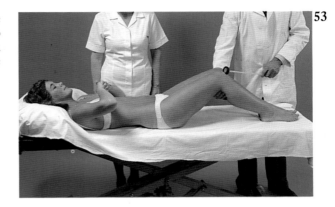

55 An alternative method of finding the ankle reflex is to flex the knee and hip with the leg externally rotated. The examiner passively dorsiflexes the patient's foot and strikes the Achilles tendon with the hammer.

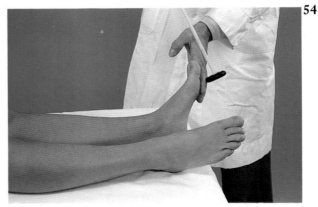

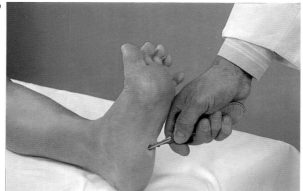

56 The plantar response is elicited with a key stroked firmly up the lateral border of the sole of the foot. This is an extensor response with the big toe extending. This indicates an upper motor neurone lesion.

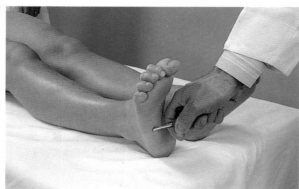

57 A flexor response is normal.

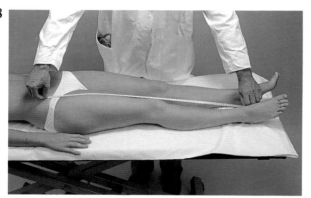

58 Leg length measurement. Some patients with sciatica cannot relax their paraspinal muscle spasm and must lie with their spine still scoliotic. This can give an impression of leg inequality; it is convenient to measure the patient before she turns face down. True length is measured from the lower edge of the anterior superior iliac spine to the lower tip of the medial malleolus. If there is a deformity of the hip or knee, each leg must be held in an equivalent position by an assistant.

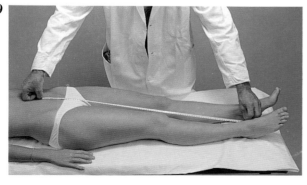

59 Apparent lengths are measured from the umbilicus to the tip of the medial malleolus. Abduction of the hip gives apparent lengthening and adduction apparent shortening. Apparent lengths are unequal sometimes when a patient cannot relax a secondary scoliosis.

60 Compression of pelvis when the patient turns on her side may cause localised pain at the site of injury, infection or neoplasia, i.e. pubic symphysis, sacroiliac joint, greater trochanter.

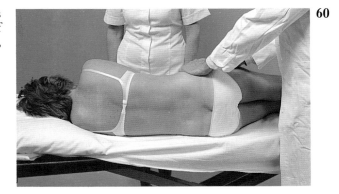

61 A demonstration of Gaenslen's test for sacroiliac stability performed on the side. On the non-examined side the hip is fully flexed and on the examined side the hip is extended (vide supra).

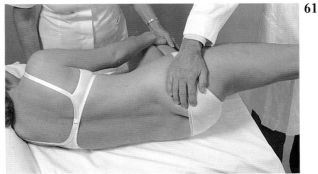

62 The power of abduction of the hip can be tested on the side (L5 root). Normal power is shown by the ability to lift the leg upwards against resistance from the examiner's hand at the knee or at the ankle.

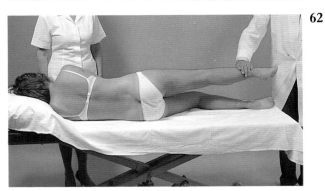

63 Lying prone, the patient's spine can be more easily palpated—first the prominent parts of the skeleton, the iliac crests, the posterior aspects of the sacroiliac joints and the lumbar spinous processes. Because the patient cannot retreat beneath the examiner's hand as when standing, more accurate delineation of tender parts can be achieved. Fixed flexion of the hip(s) will prevent the patient bringing the front of the pelvis in contact with the couch.

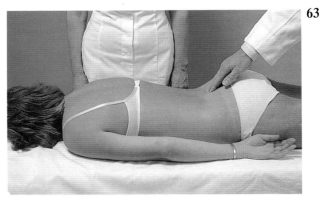

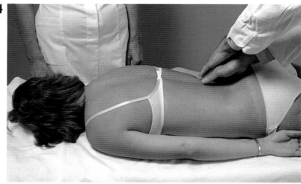

64 Deep palpation in the loin may elicit tenderness arising from the region of the transverse processes or from the kidney.

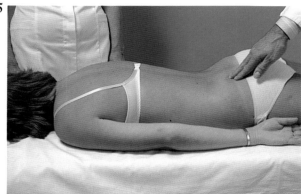

65 Palpation of the paramedian tissues may detect tenderness in the muscles or very occasionally tenderness in the sacroiliac joint.

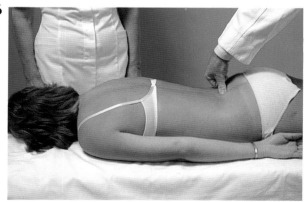

66 Deep pressure over a spinous process or interspinous ligament may elicit localised pain and reveal the chief site of instability. A step in the line of the spinous processes may be a sign of spondylolisthesis (usually at L5/S1 or L4/5).

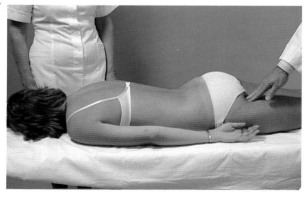

67 Palpation in the buttock at the lower edge of gluteus maximus may elicit tenderness in the sciatic nerve or cause referred pain lower down the leg.

68 Femoral nerve stretch tests. The femoral nerve passes in front of the hip joint and is stretched by hip extension with or without knee flexion. It is important to differentiate pain produced by stretching fixed flexion of the hip, but this abnormality should have been detected when the patient was supine. If there is no fixed flexion and the patient can lie prone without pain, passive knee flexion may reproduce pain in the front of the thigh and the medial aspect of the knee.

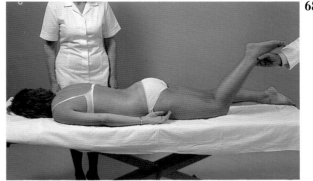

69 The femoral nerve can also be stretched by passively extending the hip.

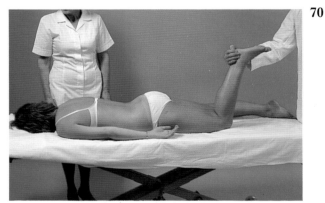

70 The relative strengths of the hamstring muscles can be tested with the patient face down. The patient is asked to bend the knee and pull the heel into the examiner's hand. Like other tests of strength, this is a relatively subjective test, dependent on the patient's co-operation.

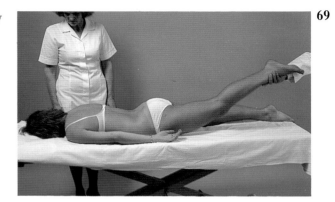

71 The gluteus maximus makes up most of the bulk of the buttock and its chief nerve supply is from the first sacral root. Weakness can be detected readily by asking the patient to squeeze the buttocks together or extend the hip. Paralysis for more than a month results in visible wasting of the buttock(s).

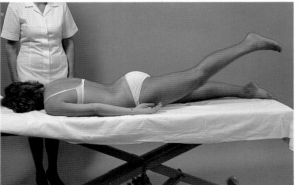

72

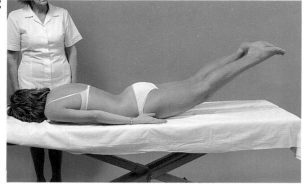

72 The power of the spinal and hip extensors is tested by asking the patient to lift both knees together off the couch. However, this action may be inhibited by lack of hip or spinal extension.

73

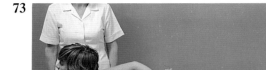

73 Spinal extensor power can also be tested by lifting the head and shoulders with the arms behind the back.

74

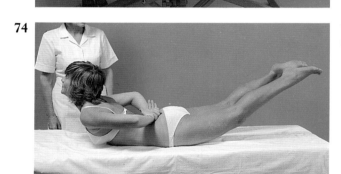

74 Strong patients can lift shoulders and legs simultaneously.

75

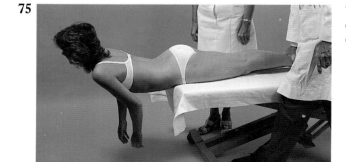

75 Athletic patients without any spinal pathology can perform unsupported spinal extension over the end of a couch.

76 Rectal examination. This step is the last part of the physical examination and can be combined with a further examination of the genitalia. The patient lies on his side with the underclothes removed and the knees drawn up. The examiner wears a glove and, if right handed, has the patient lying on his left side. The upper buttock is drawn upwards and the perineum is inspected. The tone and sensitivity of the anal sphincter is noted. Within the rectum the walls are palpated on each side as high as the examiner's finger will reach. The lumen, the walls and the structures outside the wall should be considered. In men the prostate and seminal vesicles and in women the cervix and ovaries should be identified.

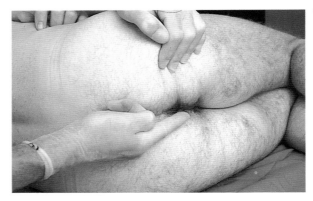

Investigations

Blood tests

The erythrocyte sedimentation rate (ESR) is a rapid test that can often differentiate menopausal osteoporosis from myelomatosis or spinal osteitis from metastases. The normal fall in 1 hour is 5-15 mm. Very high levels are recorded in severe chronic infection, rheumatoid arthritis, myelomatosis and leukaemia.

A full blood count is useful in differentiating anaemia, infections or metastases which may affect the spinal column.

A biochemical profile provides information on the calcium, phosphate, alkaline phosphatase and prostate specific antigen levels which are sometimes vital in the investigation of metabolic bone disease and neoplasia.

Rarely, other tests will help to clarify more obscure causes of low back pain, i.e. Rheumatoid Factor, HLA-27 for ankylosing spondylitis, Brucella and Salmonella titres for obscure osteitis.

Radiographic investigations

In many cases of low back pain the diagnosis rests on the radiographs; good films are essential in all cases.

The anteroposterior view of the lumbar spine should show L1 to at least the upper margin of the sacroiliac joints (S1). While inspecting the films the observer should look for a straight spine and side-to-side symmetry. The number of lumbar type vertebrae should be counted. The bones can be examined first by checking the transverse processes, the pedicles, the spinous processes and then the vertebral bodies. The disc spaces are more difficult to define and are better seen in the lateral view. The sacroiliac joints may be asymmetrical by reason of lumbosacral segmentation anomalies. Abnormalities of the sacroiliac joints are best reviewed in the appropriate left and right oblique films.

The soft tissues should next be inspected. The shadows of psoas major muscle are usually visible and should be symmetrical. Calcified lesions outside the skeleton should be noted and compared with their position on the lateral projection films.

The lateral films of the lumbar spine are particularly useful for showing the upper 4 lumbar discs and lumbar vertebral bodies. The disc spaces should gradually increase in depth from above downwards. In the young spine the lumbar vertebral bodies should be of even density. Usually the spinous processes have to be inspected against a bright light, because they are only faintly visible on a conventional screen.

The lumbosacral disc space, so often the site of pathology, is not well shown on a large plate illustrating the other lumbar disc spaces. This is because the xray beam centred on L2/3 strikes the edges of the plate at an oblique angle. Better films are obtained by centring the beam on the lumbosacral space. The exposure is also improved as allowance can be made for the overlying iliac crests. The depth of the lumbosacral disc should be equal to or larger than that of the L4/5 space above. However, if there is an associated segmentation anomaly, the lumbosacral disc will be less in depth than the L4/5 disc throughout life.

Oblique views of the lumbar spine are useful to show the posterior intervertebral joints and will show the pars interarticularis between the superior and inferior facets of each vertebral body. Left and right projections are required to show each side of the spine.

Oblique views of the sacrum will show the sacroiliac joints in profile. They are mandatory if local osteitis or ankylosing spondylitis is suspected.

Discography

For a discogram the partly sedated patient lies on his side under the image intensifiers. Local anaesthetic (10 ml 0.5 percent prilocaine) is injected into the flank.

After 2-3 minutes a spinal needle is introduced down the same track and is introduced into the centre of the disc under the control of the image intensifiers. It is important to avoid the cauda equina or the emergent nerve roots. The patient will be able to report pain in the leg if this occurs. 1-2 ml of radio-opaque water soluble contrast is injected when it is certain that the tip of the needle is in the centre of the nucleus pulposus. If the disc is normal it is difficult to inject even as much as 0.5 ml of contrast. If it is abnormal, 2 ml will go in with minimal pressure.

A normal discogram shows the contrast medium lying discretely in the centre of the disc—a 'bun' image.

A double 'bun' or 'hamburger' image indicates early degenerative changes.

A definitely abnormal disc is shown up by contrast spreading horizontally in the disc space or even leaking into the spinal canal.

A degenerative disc may not be the chief site of the patient's pain. In all patients any pain from the procedure should be interpreted with reserve and in the light of the history and physical examination.

Computerised axial tomography

Computerised axial tomography (CT scans) have become available in the past 10 years. They have proved to be a valuable aid in defining the exact cause of symptoms in patients whose problems have not been solved by more conventional methods. Very exact delineation of the skeletal and soft-tissue anatomy at the lumbosacral level is now possible. CT scans are required in only a minority of cases but patients are required to lie perfectly still for 5 minutes while being irradiated by minute doses of xrays. It is also an advantage if they are not claustrophobic, because they are surrounded by machinery during this time. The more modern machines can now differentiate between the bone of the spinal canal and the various soft-tissue structures within, but may not equal the definition of modern nuclear magnetic resonance imaging (NMRI).

Nuclear magnetic resonance imaging

NMRI is the latest tool to unravel the details of abnormal anatomy in the lumbar spine. Like CT scanning it is expensive and non-invasive but seems better at demonstrating the soft tissues. The technique and interpretation are still developing. Sections in the sagittal and transverse planes are particularly useful for showing lumbar stenosis, herniation of the nucleus pulposus and nerve root entrapment. Nerve roots and extra dural fat can be seen clearly.

The chief contraindications are the presence of cardiac pacemakers or other metallic foreign bodies within the trunk. Restlessness or claustrophobia are relative contraindications which can usually be overcome.

Lumbar puncture and lumbar myelography

A lumbar puncture will allow examination of the cerebrospinal fluid (CSF) and measurement of the pressure within the spinal canal. A raised pressure is indicative of infection or a blockage. Usually the procedure is combined with a myelogram (contraindicated if an infection or raised intracranial pressure is suspected).

The patient lies on his side with the knees drawn up to flex the lumbar spine as far as possible. The pelvis and shoulder should be in the vertical plane so that no rotation is present. The skeletal protuberances are palpated to define the position of the posterior superior iliac spines and the L5 and S1 spinous processes.

5 ml of local anaesthetic is injected into the skin and interspinous ligament at the L5/S1 or L4/5 interval: whichever seems most appropriate or easiest of access.

After 2-3 minutes a long thin spinal needle with stilette is introduced into the interspinous ligament at right angles to the coronal and sagittal plane and perpendicular to the skin. The needle must be inserted in the midline to tap the CSF and to avoid the nerve roots just lateral to the midline. A characteristic 'give' is felt as the point of the needle penetrates the ligamentum flavum and the dura mater.

The stilette is withdrawn and a drop of CSF should appear. The manometer and three-way tap are fitted to the needle and the pressure of CSF is measured. If a spinal block is suspected, Queckenstedt's test of jugular compression is performed by an assistant. If there is no obstruction to the circulation of CSF, there is a rapid rise of pressure.

After the pressure is measured, the CSF in the manometer is allowed to run into two sterile universal containers for laboratory investigations. If more CSF is required, this can be obtained by turning the three-way tap.

Qualities of cerebrospinal fluid (CSF)

Normally CSF is crystal clear. If red, the blood has usually been introduced by perforating a blood vessel when inserting the needle but a subarachnoid haemorrhage will also cause blood staining.

If yellow, there may be an obstruction to CSF circulation or an old subarachnoid haemorrhage or the patient may be jaundiced (xanthochromia).

Normal CSF pressure is 50-150 mm of water when the patient lies horizontally. CSF glucose level is below plasma level although varying with the plasma levels. It is low in bacterial meningitis.

Normal CSF contains a few cells—monocytes and leucocytes.

A lymphocytosis is found in viral meningitis and encephalitis, TB, meningitis and neurosyphilis. A leucocytosis is present in bacterial meningitis.

CSF protein levels rise in many neurological diseases. It is particularly high in a complete spinal block, in neurofibromas and in Guillain-Barré polyneuropathy.

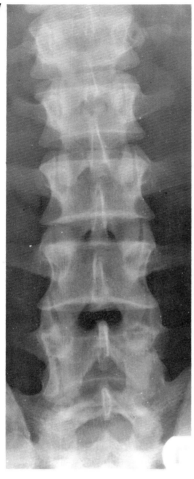

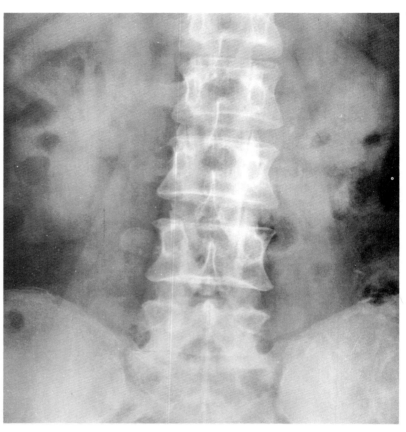

77 Xrays. In many cases of low back pain the diagnosis rests on the radiographs and good films are essential in all cases. The anteroposterior view of the normal lumbar spine should show L1 to at least the upper margin of the sacroiliac joints (S1). While inspecting the films the observer should look for a straight spine and side-to-side symmetry. The number of lumbar type vertebrae should be counted. The bones can be examined by checking the transverse processes, the pedicles, the spinous processes and then the bodies. The disc spaces are more difficult to check and are better seen in the lateral view. The sacroiliac joints may be asymmetrical by reason of lumbosacral segmentation anomalies. Abnormalities of the sacroiliac joints are best reviewed in the appropriate left and right oblique films.

78 An anteroposterior view of the lumbar spine showing the outline of psoas major muscle. The soft tissues should be inspected. The shadows of psoas major are usually visible and should be symmetrical. Asymmetry or a bulging or an obliterated margin may be caused by an infection, haematoma or neoplasm. Calcified lesions outside the skeleton should be noted and compared with their position on the lateral projection films.

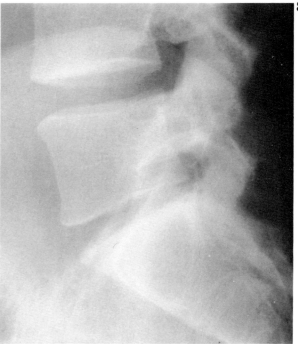

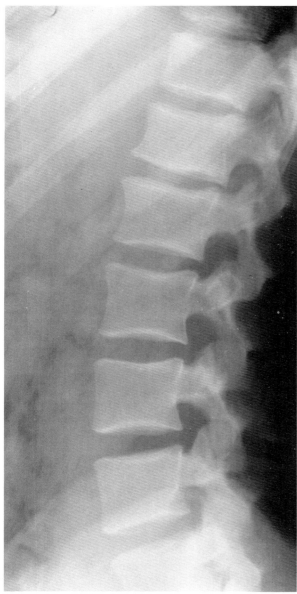

80 A lateral view of a normal lumbosacral angle: the lumbosacral disc space, so often the site of pathology, is not well shown on a large plate illustrating the other lumbar disc spaces. This is because the xray beam centred on L2/3 strikes the edges of the plate at an oblique angle. Better films are obtained by centring the beam on the lumbosacral space. The exposure is also better as due allowance can be made for the overlying iliac crests. The depth of the lumbosacral disc should be equal to or larger than that of the L4/5 space above. However, if there is an associated segmentation anomaly, the lumbosacral disc will be less in depth than the L4/5 disc throughout life.

79 The lateral film of the normal lumbar spine: this is particularly useful for showing the upper 4 lumbar discs and lumbar vertebral bodies. The disc spaces should gradually increase in depth from above downwards. In the young spine the lumbar vertebral bodies are free of osteophytes and in all spinal columns the vertebral bodies should be of even density. Usually the spinous processes have to be inspected against a bright light as they are only faintly visible on a conventional screen.

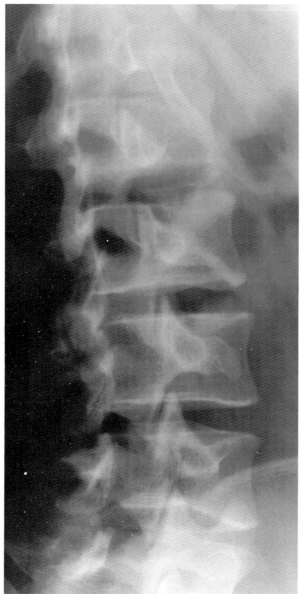

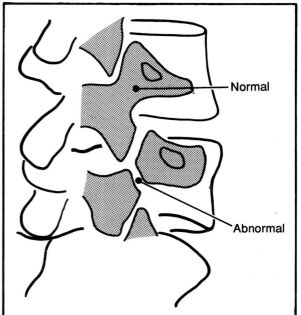

82 Diagram showing an oblique radiographic view of the lumbar spine: with a normal and a separated pars intra-articularis.

81 Oblique views of the lumbar spine to show the normal posterior intervertebral joints. The pars intra-articularis between the superior and inferior facets of each vertebral body is well seen. Left and right projections are required to show each side of the spine.

Oblique views of the sacrum will show the sacroiliac joints in profile. They are mandatory if local osteitis or ankylosing spondylitis is suspected.

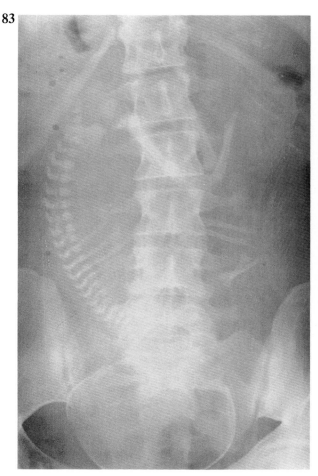

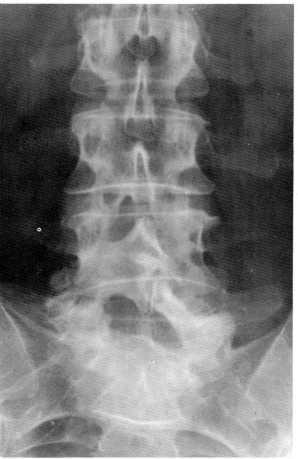

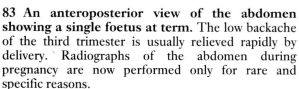

83 An anteroposterior view of the abdomen showing a single foetus at term. The low backache of the third trimester is usually relieved rapidly by delivery. Radiographs of the abdomen during pregnancy are now performed only for rare and specific reasons.

84 Spina bifida is an embryological defect caused by the failure of closure of the neural tube in the first weeks after conception. The more gross examples are incompatible with life but the minor defects lower in the lumbar region are sometimes free of neurological lesions. In between are a wide range of abnormalities resulting in spinal deformity and varying neurological defects. In the more minor conditions, the only clues to underlying skeletal changes may be a midline skin dimple or an isolated patch of hair.

The most minor skeletal abnormality may be a midline gap in the neural arch seen on the anteroposterior films at L5 or S1, as shown in the illustration. Usually no neural or meningeal abnormality is present and the overlying skin is normal. Such midline neural arch defects are not productive of backache unless there are associated anomalies of the transverse processes or intervertebral disc.

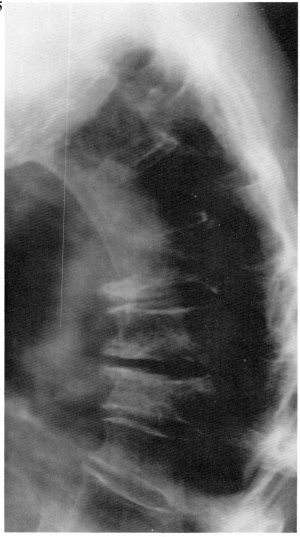

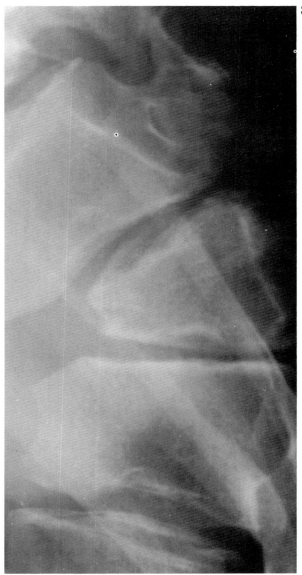

85 A lateral view of the thoracic spine showing a congenital fusion of three upper thoracic vertebral bodies.

Congenital fusion of vertebra either at the bodies or neural arches or both may give rise to a stiff segment and premature degenerative changes at the mobile joints, immediately above and below the fused segment. Unilateral or asymmetric fusion will cause a congenital kyphoscoliosis.

86 A lateral radiograph of the lower thoracic spine to show a kyphus caused by congenital malformation of a vertebral body. This gives a localised fixed segment. By middle-age there will be arthritic changes in the nearby joints. Other causes of a short segment kyphus are trauma, infection and neoplasia.

87 Anterolateral radiograph of the lumbosacral junction showing asymmetry of segmentation in the transverse processes. Sacralisation of the 5th lumbar vertebra can be unilateral or bilateral. The unilateral forms give rise to asymmetrical spinal movement and are frequently associated with low back pain in early adult life, especially if the patient engages in strenuous work or vigorous sport.

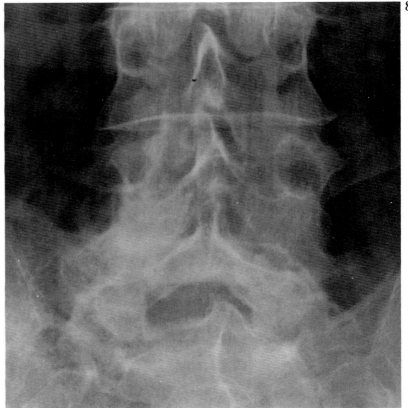

88 An anteroposterior radiographic view of the lumbosacral junction showing partial sacralisation of L5—the transverse processes articulate with the ilium.

Segmentation anomalies are extremely common at the lumbosacral level but it is uncertain whether the total number of vertebral bodies in the individual spinal column is altered. Four or six lumbar vertebrae instead of the usual five is said to increase the likelihood of low back pain, prolapsed intervertebral disc or localised degenerative change. Above and below the thoracic region of the spinal column anomalies of the ribs are often seen, i.e. cervical or lumbar ribs unilaterally and bilaterally.

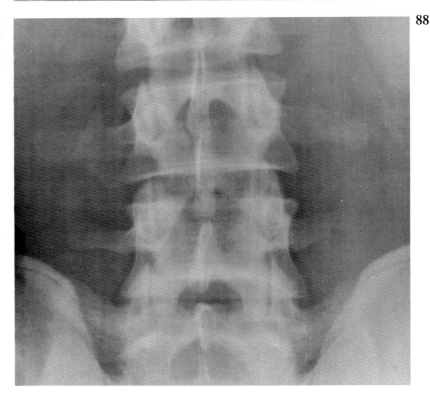

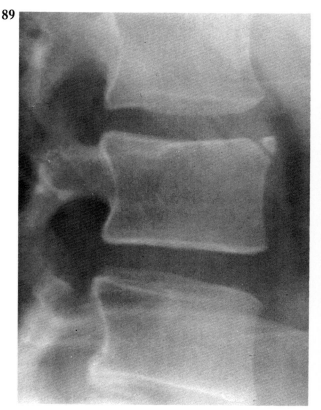

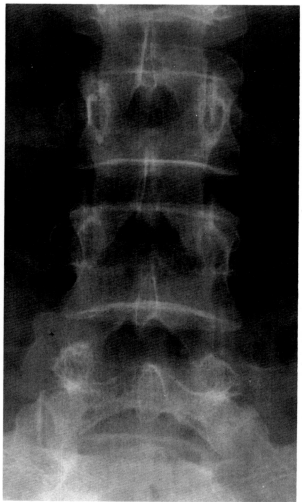

89 A lateral view of the mid-lumbar spine showing failure of fusion of a ring epiphysis at the upper anterior margin of a vertebral body.

The adolescent ring epiphyses of the lumbar vertebrae may fail to fuse at the anterior angles of the vertebral bodies. The radiographs suggest a possible fracture but a history of injury is usually lacking and there is no other radiological sign of injury. It is doubtful if such a failure of fusion is itself a cause of low back pain, unless several vertebral bodies are affected.

90 An anteroposterior view of the lumbosacral junction showing asymmetry of the lower two sets of posterior facet joints, compared to the normal appearance of the upper two sets of joints. Asymmetry of the posterior facet joints is quite common at the L5/S1 level and less often at the L4/5 level. It may be a hidden cause of low back pain of mechanical origin. There may be an associated segmentation anomaly as well.

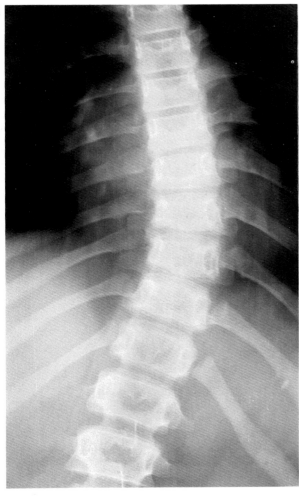

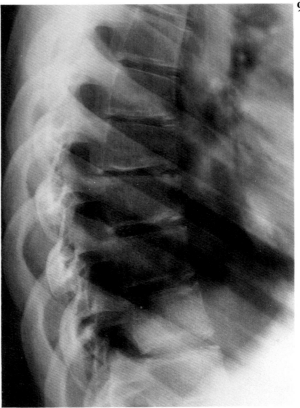

92 A lateral view of the thoracic spine showing irregular ossification of the anterior parts of the ring epiphyses of the vertebral bodies.

91 An anteroposterior view of the lower thoracic spine showing a moderate scoliosis. A scoliosis is a lateral curvature of the spine in the coronal plane. There are many causes apart from hemivertebrae, etc. Usually there is a smooth curvature extending over several vertebrae. Fractures, neoplasms or localised infections may give a short angular curvature.

If a scoliosis exists for many years, then degenerative changes develop in the adjacent joints and a previously painless curve becomes painful.

A long high thoracic kyphosis in late adolescence or early adult life without a scoliosis or any history of trauma may be caused by an epiphysitis affecting the ring epiphyses of the vertebral bodies, which are present at the margins of the vertebral bodies in the teens. The cause of the irregular ossification is not known, but the effect is to produce a wedging of the vertebral bodies and an obvious round-shouldered appearance (Scheuermann's disease). The condition usually affects tall young males with tight hamstrings. Backache does not often accompany the physical appearance.

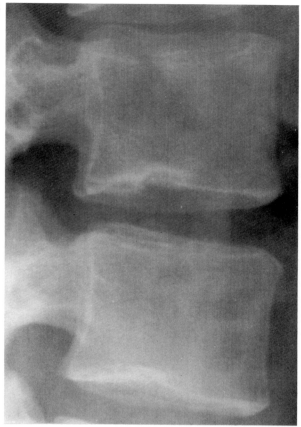

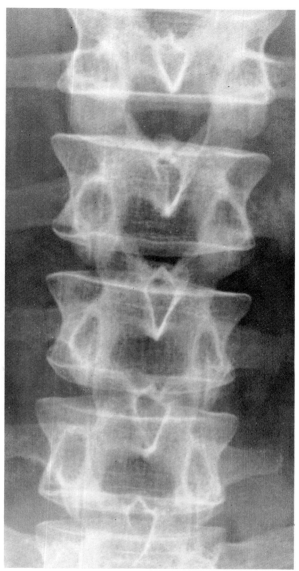

93 A lateral view of the mid-lumbar spine to show a small central disc protrusion into the body of the vertebra above. Early degenerative changes in an intervertebral disc may be first seen on radiographs as a central protrusion of disc substance into the end plate of the adjacent vertebral body (Schmorl's nodes). This usually occurs before any loss of disc height or before any posterior or posterolateral protrusion produces low back pain. Schmorl's nodes may be present at several levels. It is doubtful if they produce any symptoms in themselves, especially in the early stages of development.

94 An anteroposterior view of L3 lumbar spine to show an undisplaced fracture of the right transverse process. This occurs from an injury and gives rise to unilateral backache without sciatica. Pain improves steadily over several weeks.

95 A lateral view of the lumbar spine showing a healing compression fracture of a vertebral body. This will cause a localised kyphus posteriorly and very long continued backache.

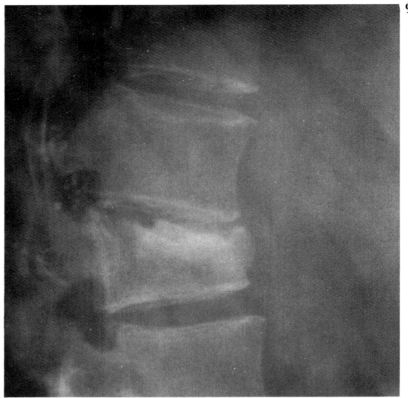

96 A lateral tomographic view of the lower thoracic spine showing erosion of adjacent margins of the vertebral bodies. Infection of a disc space produces loss of space between the adjacent vertebral bodies and rarefaction of the adjacent vertebral end plates.

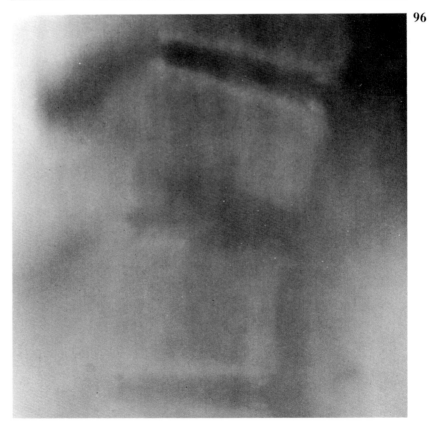

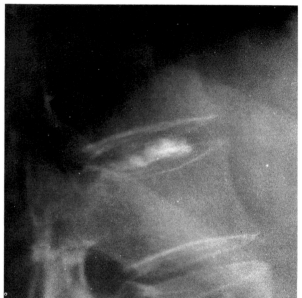

97 A lateral view of the lumbar spine showing calcification of a disc. This is said to be caused by a localised infection but this is doubtful. It produces acute pain which may resolve after some months. The radiological changes may fade later.

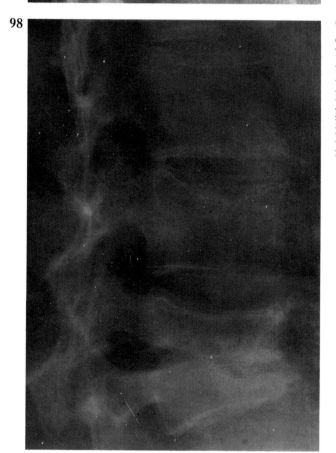

98 A lateral view of the lumbar spine showing collapse and fusion of L2 and L3 vertebral bodies. There is irregular calcification anteriorly in the abdomen. Tuberculous osteitis of the spine usually originates in the vertebral body end plate leading to local rarefaction and erosion of the end plate. The disc space is eventually obliterated and the local vertebral bodies become wedge shaped. A local kyphus develops and, in untreated cases, paraplegia may follow.

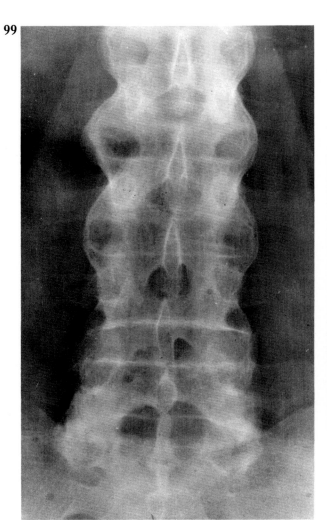

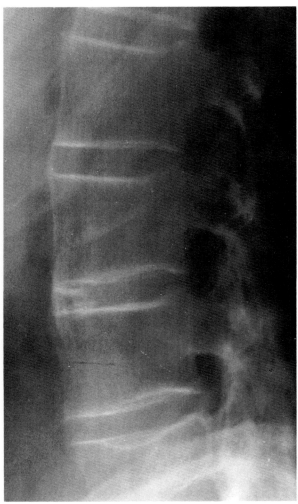

99 An anteroposterior view of the lumbar spine in ankylosing spondylitis. There is ossification of the paraspinal ligaments (bamboo spine).

100 Lateral view of the lumbar spine in ankylosing spondylitis. There is squaring of the vertebral bodies and ossification in the anterior longitudinal ligament.

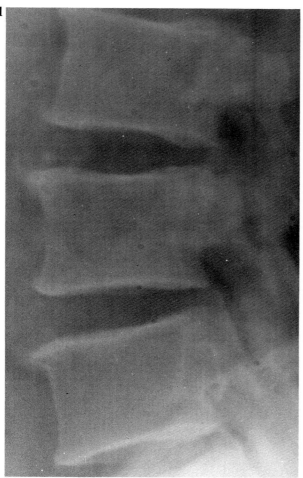

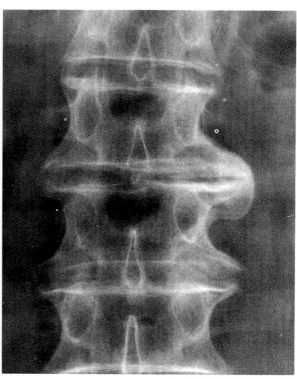

102 Anteroposterior view of the lumbar spine showing a large lateral osteophyte that virtually unites the adjacent vertebral bodies. Other osteophytes are also visible.

101 Lateral view of the lumbar spine shows early degenerative changes at 3 disc levels. There are small osteophytes at the anterior angles of the vertebral bodies.

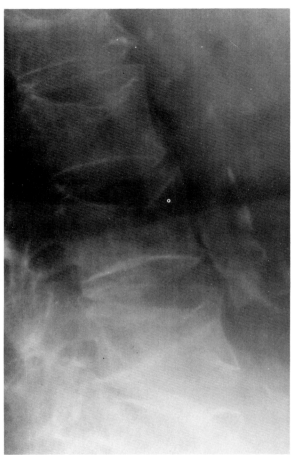

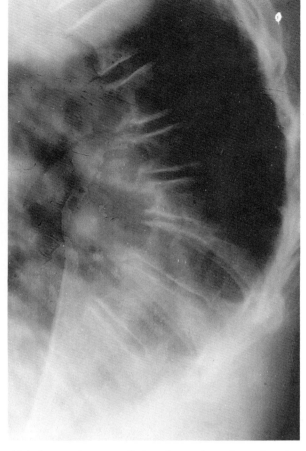

**103 Lateral view of the lumbar spine showing
osteoporotic compression** of several vertebral
bodies. The enlargement of the disc spaces deforms
the vertebral bodies ('fish-tailed vertebrae').

**104 Lateral view of the thoracic spine showing
a kyphus** caused by wedged vertebral bodies. There
are degenerative changes above and below the apical
vertebrae.

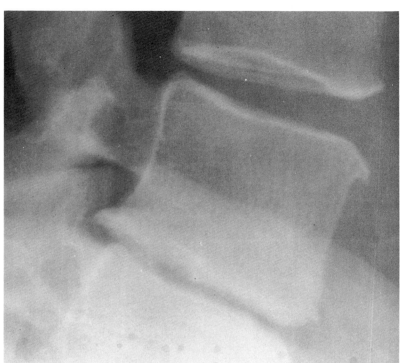

105 Lateral view of the lumbar spine showing marked degeneration of the lower disc space with loss of height and a posterior osteophyte. There is likely to be pain and a neurological deficit in the nerve roots emergent at this level.

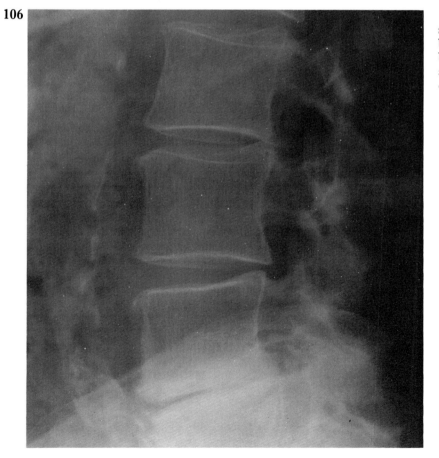

106 Lateral view of the lumbar spine showing disc degeneration between **L4 and L5** and also between L5 and S1. The abdominal aorta is calcified and dilated opposite L2 and L3.

107 Lateral view of the lumbar spine to show a forward slip of one vertebra on the one beneath. This is caused by the defect in the neural arch which is visible posteriorly (spondylolisthesis).

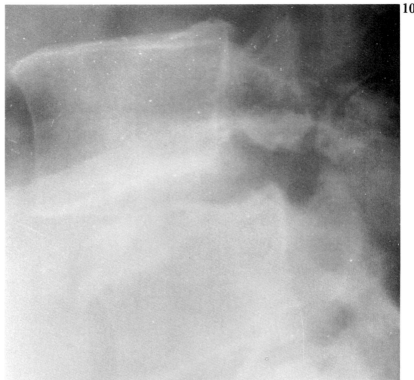

108 Lateral view of the lumbar spine showing a gross spondylolisthesis of L3 on L4. This is caused by an old fatigue fracture of the neural arch at the pars intra-articularis. L3 moves forwards dragging on the emergent L3 roots at the L3/4 interspace. There may be pain and a neurological deficit.

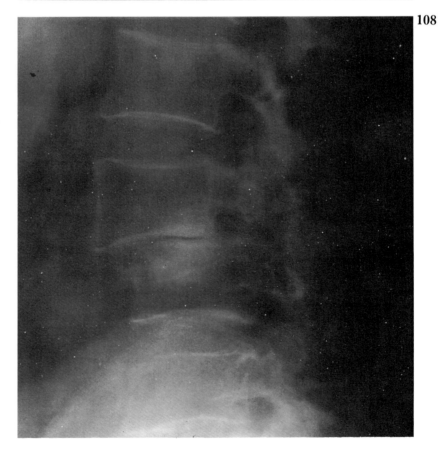

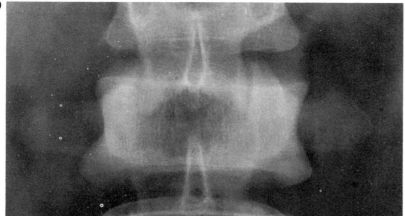

109 Anteroposterior view of the lumbar spine showing a solitary dense vertebra. This is usually caused by a prostatic metastases or Paget's disease and often produces low grade unremitting backache.

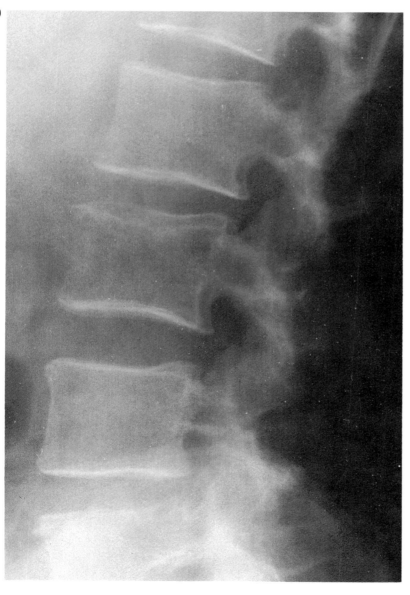

110 Lateral view of the lumbar spine showing erosion of the anterior margin of the third lumbar vertebral body from a secondary deposit of a carcinoma of the breast. This produces severe, rapidly worsening backache, which may progress to paraplegia.

111 Lateral view of the lumbar spine and abdomen. The diffuse calcification anterior to L2 lies in the pancreas and is a sign of chronic pancreatitis. Backache is not always present.

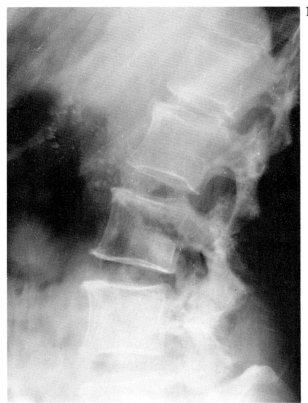

112 Anteroposterior view of the lumbar spine showing an abdominal aortic aneurysm. This is an xray of an old person showing a rim of calcified material lateral to the spine on one side. The calcification in the iliac vessels is visible below. An intravenous pyelogram has been performed, but only one kidney is visualised. Backache of a severe unremitting character is usually present but no sciatica. The legs may be ischaemic.

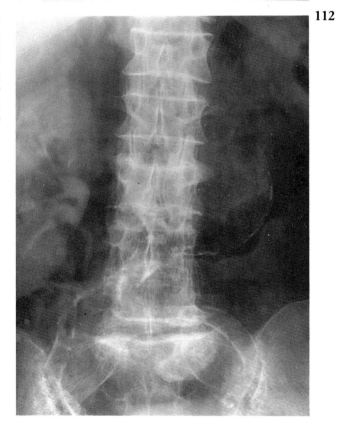

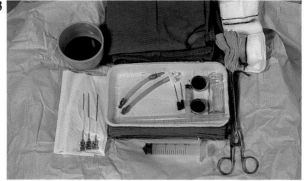

113 **A lumbar puncture** will allow examination of CSF and measurement of the pressure within the spinal canal. A raised pressure is indicative of infection or a blockage. Usually the procedure is combined with a myelogram. A lumbar puncture is contraindicated if there is a suspicion of raised intracranial pressure. A myelogram is contraindicated if an infection is present or suspected.

Materials for lumbar puncture:

- Small sterile dressing pack
- 1 per cent iodine in spirit
- Sponge holders
- Gallipot
- Local anaesthetic
- 10 ml syringe and needles
- CSF manometer
- Three-way tap
- Connecting tubing
- Universal containers

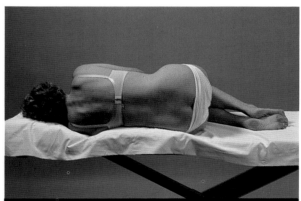

114 **The patient lies on her side with the knees drawn up** to flex the lumbar spine as far as possible. The pelvis and shoulders should be in the vertical plane so that no rotation is present. The skeletal protuberances are palpated and marked to define the position of the posterior superior iliac spines and the L5 and S1 spinous processes.

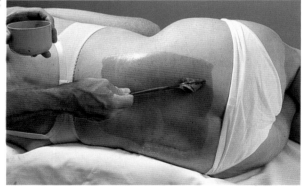

115 **Skin preparation with 1 per cent iodine in spirit** (provided there is no sensitivity to iodine). Hibitane in spirit is an alternative antiseptic.

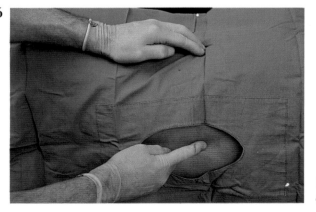

116 **Towels are draped** over the patient and the correct interspinous gap is palpated.

117 5 ml of local anaesthetic is injected into the skin and interspinous ligament at the L5/S1 or L4/5 interval. Either is suitable depending on whichever is appropriate or easiest of access.

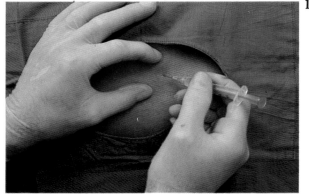

118 A long thin spinal needle with a stillete introduced into the interspinous ligament 2-3 minutes after the injection of local anaesthetic.

The needle must be at right angles to the coronal and sagittal planes and perpendicular to the skin. The needle must be inserted in the midline to tap the CSF and to avoid the nerve roots just lateral to the midline. A characteristic 'give' is felt as the point of the needle penetrates the ligamentum flavum and dura mater.

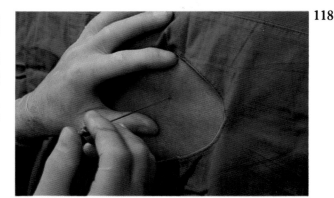

119 The stillete is withdrawn and a drop of CSF should appear. The manometer and three-way tap is fitted to the needle and the pressure of CSF is measured.

If a spinal block is suspected, Queckenstedt's test of jugular compression is performed by an assistant. If there is no obstruction to the circulation of CSF, there is a rapid rise of CSF pressure.

With the pressure measured, the CSF in the manometer is allowed to run off into two sterile universal containers for laboratory investigations. If more CSF is required, this can be obtained by turning the three-way tap.

If no myelogram is to be performed, the needle is withdrawn at this stage from the patient and an adhesive dressing is applied. The patient is advised to lie flat for the next 24 hours to avoid a headache from a diminished CSF pressure.

If a myelogram is required, the lumbar puncture is performed in the Radiology Department under the image intensifiers. After CSF specimens are obtained, the radiologist injects 5-10 ml of water soluble contrast media and can watch the contrast flow up the spinal canal on the image intensifier. The patient can be tipped and rolled to outline each level

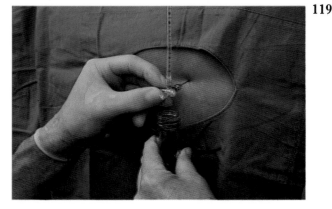

and each angle of each level to define any bulging disc or compressed nerve root. At the completion of the radiological examination, the needle is withdrawn and a small adhesive dressing applied to the puncture hole. The patient is advised to sit up for 4 hours to prevent contrast entering the head during absorption and then to lie flat for 24 hours.

Materials for myelography are usually available in a pre-sterilised pack. They are the same as for a lumbar puncture, with the addition of contrast medium.

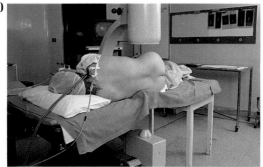

120 Discograms can be performed with sedation under image intensifiers. The patient is positioned as for a lumbar puncture. The skeletal landmarks are identified and the image intensifiers are checked for position and imaging.

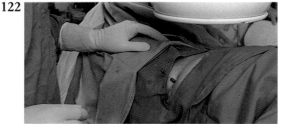

121 Local anaesthetic is injected posterolaterally in the line of the sacroiliac joint and introduced inwards towards the disc to be injected.

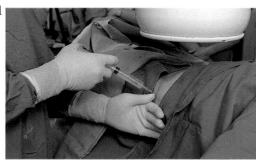

122 Using the image intensifiers a long thin spinal needle is introduced down the same track and passed into the centre of the appropriate disc. It is important to avoid penetrating the spinal canal or the spinal dura.

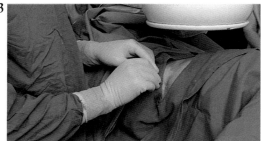

123 The position of the needle is adjusted so that the tip lies centrally in the disc.

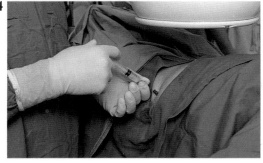

124 If a discogram is required, 1-2 ml of contrast medium is then injected. Alternatively if disc shrinkage is indicated, the appropriate dose of chymopapein is injected. The two substances are never injected at the same procedure. The needle is then withdrawn and a small dressing applied to the puncture hole.

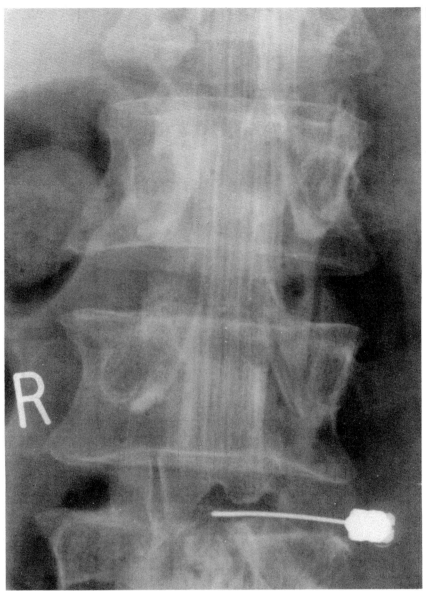

125 An anteroposterior view of the lower lumbar spine showing the cauda equina outlined by water soluble contrast medium injected for a lumbar myelogram.

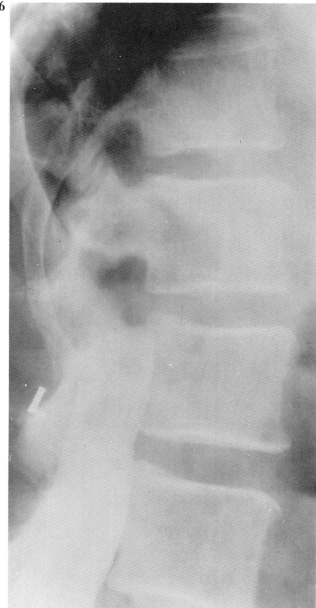

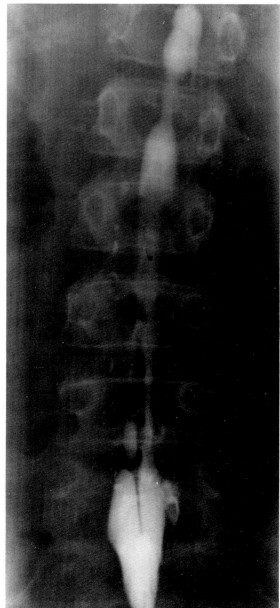

126 Lateral view of the lumbar spine showing a complete block to a column of contrast medium injected from below. This may be caused by a disc protrusion or an intrathecal tumour.

127 Anteroposterior view of the lumbar spine showing a column of contrast medium in the spinal canal. The canal is attenuated from L2 to L4 suggesting intrathecal pathology such as a secondary tumour. There is also a constriction in the spinal canal at the upper border of L1.

128 A lateral view of lumbar discograms. The upper disc injected is normal while the lower disc is abnormal, in that contrast has flowed both posteriorly and laterally.

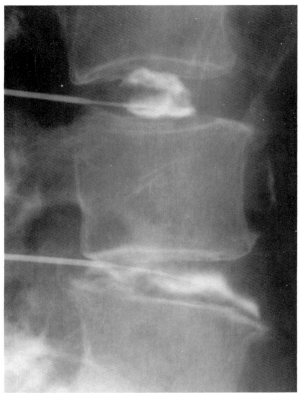

129 Oblique view of the abdomen during a barium meal. A penetrating duodenal ulcer is outlined. Such a lesion sometimes gives rise to intermittent right upper lumbar backache between meals or during the night.

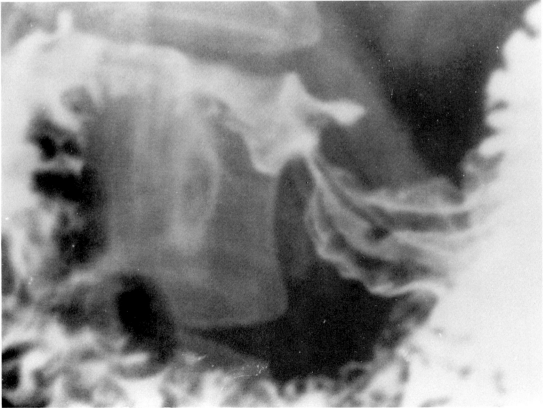

130

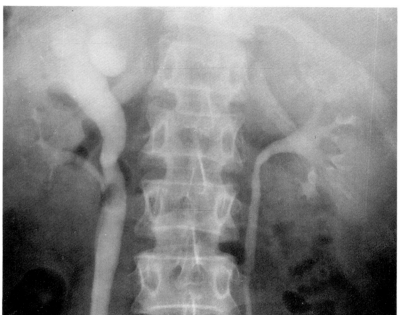

130 An intravenous pyelogram showing a hydronephrotic right kidney and a dilated ureter. This may be a cause of unilateral chronic backache situated in the loin.

131

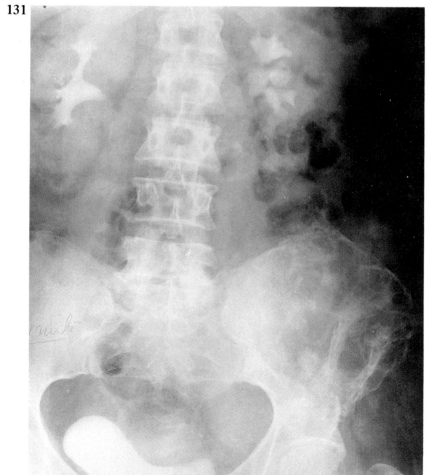

131 Anteroposterior view of the abdomen during an intravenous pyelogram. A hypernephroma of the left kidney has metastasised to the left ilium. The body of L4 is infiltrated and the bladder is indented. Such a combination of lesions is likely to cause severe unilateral backache steadily worsening. Urinary symptoms may be absent in some cases until a late stage in the disease.

132 A CT scan of the lumbosacral disc in a horizontal plane. A posterior protrusion of the disc can be seen clearly impinging in the left lateral root canal. This is likely to cause severe sciatica with a neurological defect.

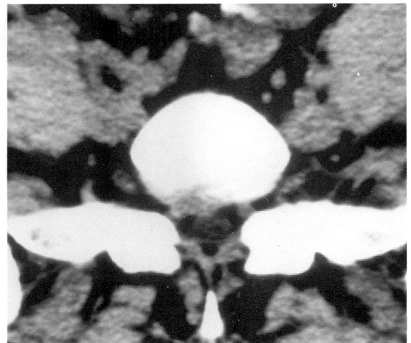

133 An NMRI of the midline sagittal plane of the lumbar spine showing the spinal canal, spinal cord, vertebral bodies and lumbar discs. There is a small posterior disc protrusion at the lumbar 4/5 level.

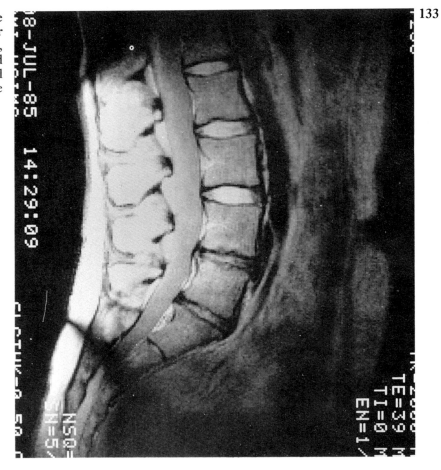

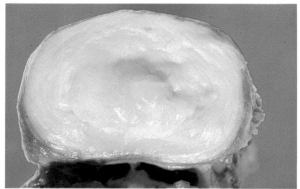

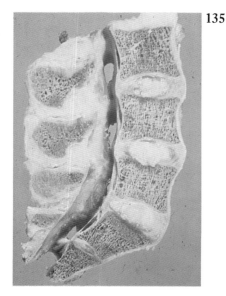

134 Horizontal transverse section through a normal human lumbar intervertebral disc. The nucleus pulposus and the outer annulus fibrosus can be seen clearly.

135 A sagittal section through the lumbar spine showing the spinal canal, vertebral bodies and the intervertebral discs.

136

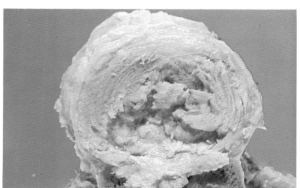

136 Horizontal transverse section through an abnormal human intervertebral disc. There is degeneration and dehydration of the nucleus pulposus and stretching of the annulus fibrosus.

137 A sagittal section through a lumbar spine showing degeneration and posterior protrusion of an intervertebral disc. This is likely to impinge on a lumbar nerve root to cause a sciatica.

137

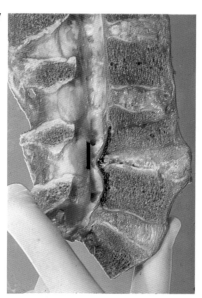

138 A dessicated prepared specimen of two lumbar vertebrae showing osteophyte formation at the margins of the vertebral bodies. The osteophytes encroach on the intervertebral foramen posteriorly, thus diminishing the space for the emerging lumbar nerve root—another cause of sciatic pain.

138

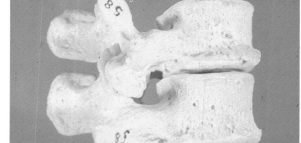

Conservative treatment

Home remedies

A soft bed will allow excessive curvature of the spine for long periods when the patient is asleep and makes turning over more difficult. A firm mattress prevents excessive curvature of the spine during sleep. A thin soft mattress can be hardened by placing a board at least 75 cm × 150 cm × 1 cm beneath it.

Patients with acutely painful spines may be relieved by lying on their sides with lumbar spine, hips and knees flexed or on their backs with pillows beneath the shins to give an equivalent position.

A soft easy chair acts like a soft mattress to increase spinal curvature and pain. A firm chair will encourage the sitter to preserve a straight vertical spine. In a phase of acute low back pain additional relief may be obtained by sitting astride the chair and resting the arms on the back. For those with a sedentary job and backache, a kneeling chair will make it possible to lean over a desk and still keep the spinal column straight.

A bad posture likely to promote backache is characterised by a long smooth thoracic kyphus and a lumbar lordosis. The head is pushed forward and the hips and knees are incompletely extended.

A good posture likely to avoid or diminish backache involves lifting the head, pulling the shoulders back, tucking in the abdomen and straightening the hips and knees.

Pulling heavy objects usually involves lumbar flexion and knee extension. Such a posture will provoke backache by stressing the posterior structures and opening up the posterior part of lumbar disc spaces. Tug-of-war teams are taught to lean back with a straight spine and apply their pull through the quadriceps acting on flexed knees. Pushing is usually easier, safer and more effective than pulling.

139 A firm chair will encourage the sitter to preserve a straight vertical spine. A soft easy chair acts like a soft mattress to increase spinal curvature and pain. During a phase of acute low back pain, additional relief may be obtained by sitting astride the chair and resting the arms on the backrest.

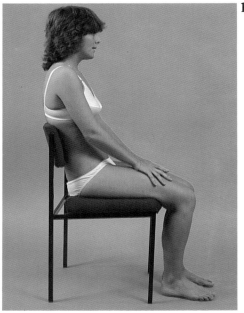

139

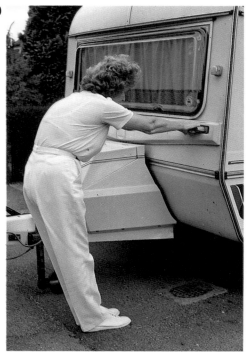 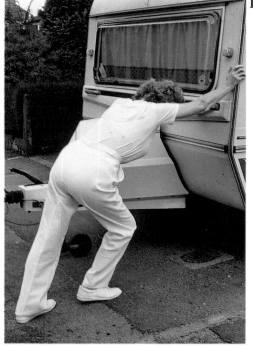

140 Pulling heavy objects usually involves lumbar flexion and knee extension. Such a posture will provoke backache by stressing the posterior structures and opening up the posterior part of lumbar disc spaces.

141 Pushing is usually easier, safer and more effective than pulling.

142

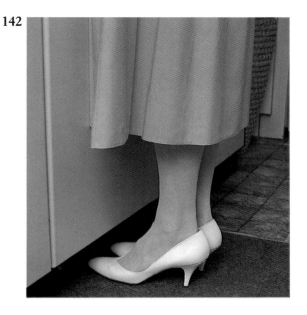

142 While standing at a bench or work-top, there is considerable relief afforded by having the toes or feet in a recess beneath the top surface. The person can stand upright and thus avoid the prolonged forward flexion which would occur if the feet were further away from the site of work.

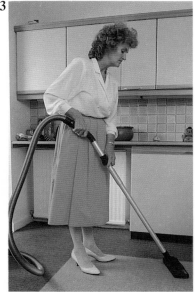

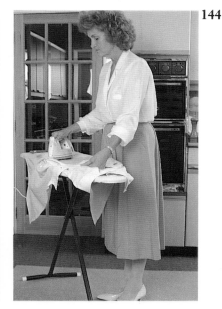

143 Long-handled tools to perform tasks at ground level while standing or walking i.e. brushes, hoes, etc. should be held near their extremities, to avoid a prolonged stooping posture.

144 Low work surfaces should be raised if possible to such a height as the person finds comfortable in either sitting or standing positions. The ironing board has been raised so that the housewife can stand up straight at her job.

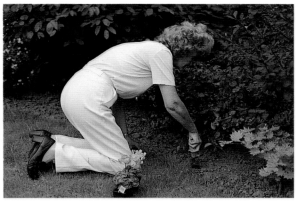

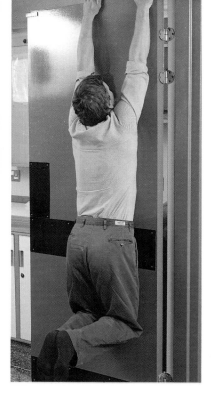

145 Gardening is a frequent cause of backache in an otherwise sedentary population. It is better to kneel down to carry out ground level jobs.

146 Temporary relief of backache is sometimes obtained by the patient applying traction to the lumbar spine by hanging by the hands off a bar or a strong door and taking the feet off the floor for a few seconds at a time. This can be repeated several times over a few minutes and the whole cycle performed several times a day. Not every patient is strong enough to perform this manoeuvre and not every patient who can will obtain relief.

Physiotherapy

In patients with musculoskeletal problems of the back, physiotherapy is often the treatment of choice. The services of a physiotherapist interested and skilled in spinal work is a great advantage. The physiotherapist will assess the patient to identify particular mechanical problems, and treatment is then aimed at correcting these. The treatment will often consist of postural and ergonomic advice, and active exercises. These will strengthen weak muscles, and stretch soft tissue and tight muscle groups. Passive accessory movements to individual vertebral joints may also be included as a part of treatment.

Pelvic tilting and spinal flattening can be practised against a wall in the standing position. This brings the lumbar spine more vertically balanced upon the pelvis. In the prone position lifting the pelvis exercises the spinal and hip extensors. Abdominal muscles are strengthened gradually by progressing from straight raising of one leg to straight raising of both legs and finally to sit up positions.

The lateral flexors of the trunk can be strengthened by the patient exercising while lying on his/her side. The uppermost leg is abducted at the hips to lift towards the ceiling. As strength improves this exercise can be performed against resistance, i.e. the therapist's hand or a weight attached to the ankle.

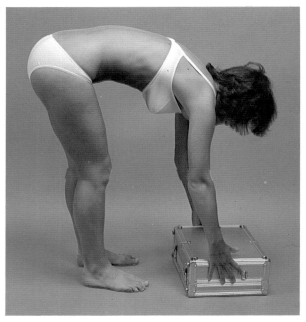

147 | **148**

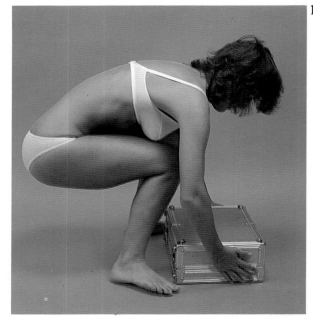

147 A bad method of lifting with the knees straight and the back bent, the maximum stress is applied to the lumbar region. This type of lifting posture should be avoided.

148 A safer method of lifting. The knees and hips are flexed to minimise the stress on the lumbar spine. When one is standing erect, the heavy object should be held close to the trunk. This is the technique of competitive weightlifters.

149 Stretching tight extensors and posterior structures can be achieved by telling the patient to hug his knees while lying supine on the couch.

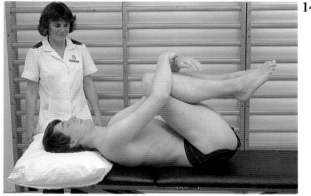

150 This is an alternative method of stretching tight extensor structures.

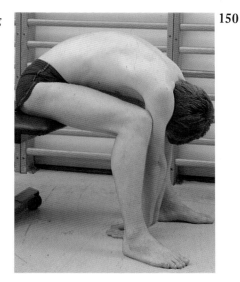

151 Stretching the necessary structures in a patient who deviates on forward flexion as a result of dysfunction can be achieved by having the patient standing with one leg on a stool. He should bend forward and reach for the elevated foot, stretching away from the side to which he deviates.

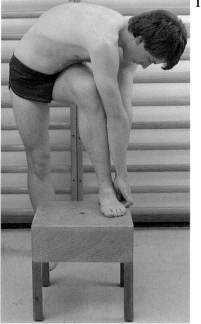

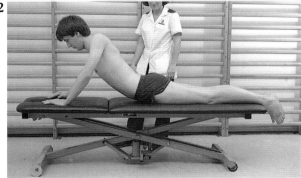

152 Stretching tight flexors and anterior structures can be achieved by getting the patient to extend his back passively.

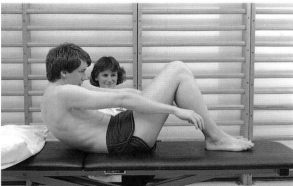

153 Strengthening of the abdominal flexor muscles is accomplished by the patient reaching with his hands to his knees and lifting his head and shoulders.

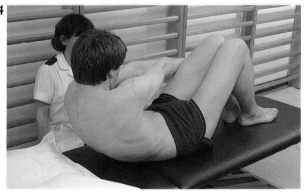

154 Unilateral exercising of abdominal flexors and stretching the opposite extensor structures is accomplished by reaching for alternative knees.

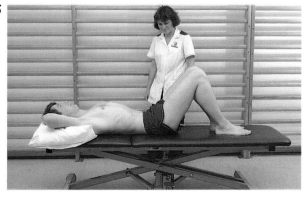

155 and 156 More abdominal strength is required for the patient in this exercise. With his lumbar spine flattened onto the couch, he straightens his knees from the flexed position, and holds both legs off the couch. This is contraindicated for patients with disc pathology.

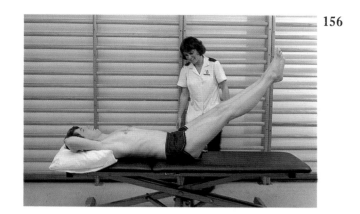

157 Strengthening of the spinal extensors is achieved by the patient lying prone and alternately lifting one leg off the bed. The leg should be kept straight.

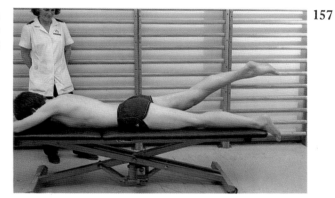

158 More spinal extensor strength is required to lift both legs together.

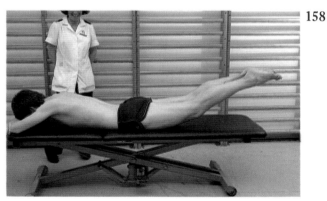

159 Even more spinal extensor strength is needed to lift legs and shoulders simultaneously.

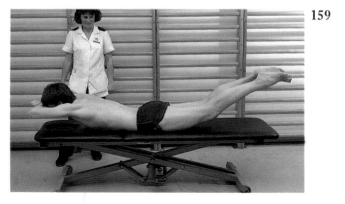

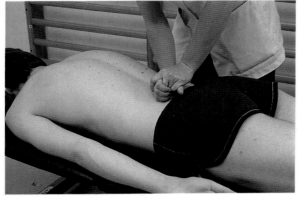

160 By careful palpation it is possible to identify individually stiff joints in the lumbar spine, and mobilise them by the use of passive accessory movements.

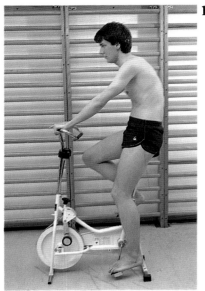

161 To complement rehabilitation of the back, leg muscles must be strengthened. Cycling both mobilises the back and strengthens the legs. Swimming is also an excellent strengthening exercise.

External splintage for low back pain

This form of treatment aims to splint the painful segment of the spine to diminish pain and to allow healing. It will fail to achieve these aims unless the patient can be accurately fitted and feels an improvement rapidly.

In adolescence the main indication is correction of a scoliosis or temporary protection of a spinal fusion. In middle life it is used for disc lesions, fractures, spondylosis and spondylolisthesis. In later life it may be considered for osteoporosis, for minor compression fractures and for degenerative changes. Relative contraindications are very thin or very fat patients. In the former, pressure points are likely to develop and in the latter, the patient's spine moves about within the coverings of soft tissue. The presence of a hiatus hernia or reduced breathing capacity is another relative contraindication, as heartburn and dyspnoea are likely to be exacerbated. The elderly are less tolerant of external splintage. They are often thin, bent and stiff, thus finding the fitting of a corset or brace distasteful and difficult. The frail elderly patient will also complain of the weight of the splint.

An elastic garment, corset or belt is the least restrictive form of external splintage but expert construction and fitting are required for comfort.

A belt or corset made from non-elastic canvas or other material may be strengthened by metal or plastic rods. This type of spinal splint is usually made to standard sizes and can be fitted quickly, if the patient is also a standard size. Unless it is a good fit, it is often uncomfortable. Made-to-measure belts take 1-2 weeks for construction and should be ordered as soon as possible. Most women, unless they are very thin, are more comfortable if they have a deep brassiere fitted at the same time as the corset and linked to it. This prevents an uncomfortable fold of flesh appearing between the top edge of the corset and the lower edge of the brassiere.

Spinal braces consist of metal frames contoured to

fit the spine, pelvis and chest and covered with leather. They give more rigid support and are put on like a coat and buckled in front. Often the straps radiate from an abdominal pad which gives extra support to the abdomen. A comfortable fit is essential. They are more expensive than corsets or belts but are more comfortable to wear in a hot climate. As they are more rigid, the bottom edge impinges on a seat so that they are pushed upwards uncomfortably if used in the sitting posture.

Even more rigid spinal support can be provided by a plastic or plaster cast or a removable plastic jacket. These are the most expensive forms of splintage and are inappropriate to hot climates. An accurate fitting is again essential. A few patients become claustrophobic in a plaster or plastic cast when they realise they cannot release themselves easily.

External splintage should be regarded as a temporary measure only. Apart from accurate fitting, its efficacy also depends on the co-operation of the patient who can wear or discard the belt at will.

External splintage worn uninterrupted for more than a few weeks leads to muscle atrophy; the patient then becomes dependent on the support. It should be made clear at the first fitting that the support will be discarded at a certain point in the near future. The patient should be taught isometric back exercises to practise with and without the support during the time it is worn. When the support is to be given up, the process should be gradual over 1-2 weeks, leaving off the support for a few hours per day at first and gradually increasing the free periods until the patient has entirely discarded it.

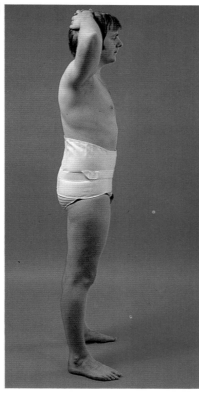

162 A lumbar belt for a man is more likely to be available 'off the shelf' in a standard design, but a good fit is still essential. More obese subjects require individual measurements and construction. The fatter the patient the less likely is a belt or corset to be capable of relieving pain.

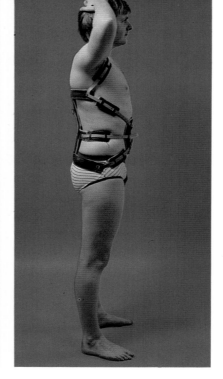

163 A brace provides a more rigid support for the lumbar and/or thoracic spine. This is made to individual measurements and requires skilled fitting. Patients should not wear such a brace for more than the prescribed period, because they can become dependent upon them.

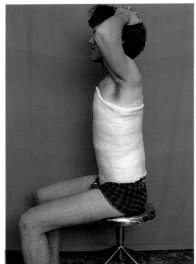

164 A plaster cast provides even more rigid external support. Although commonly applied in the recent past, these are not often used now. Skilled application is essential for comfort. Again, braces and casts are not likely to be effective in obese subjects.

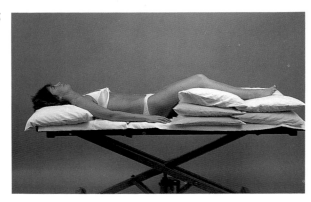

165 Patients with acutely painful spines may be relieved by lying on their sides with lumbar spine, hips and knees flexed. The equivalent position can be obtained by lying on the back with a pile of pillows under the shins.

Traction

Traction on the lumbar spine has long been used to relieve low back pain of skeletal origin. It is applied to the leg in which sciatic pain is perceived. If there is no sciatica, traction may be applied to both legs or to the pelvis. A weight of 2-3 kg can be exerted on each leg by fixation on the skin. The hairs should be shaved off. If the patient has no history of skin allergy, loops of rubberised fabric or adhesive strapping are applied to the whole length of each side of the leg from groin to ankle. The loops project beyond the foot by 15-20 cm and are bandaged onto the leg. The necessary weights are hung from the projections over the end of the bed. It is best to have the end of the bed elevated 10-15 cm and to use a pulley frame. Fragile skin and/or short legs may not accommodate more than 1-2 kg without causing discomfort or damaging the skin. Traction has the double effect of very slightly distracting the lumbar spine and splinting the overactive patient in the horizontal position.

If the state of the leg is unsuitable for traction, pelvic traction can be applied by a harness buckled around the waist. 5-7 kg can be applied in this situation but the weight is borne by the iliac crests and can become very uncomfortable unless relaxed at intervals.

In the Physiotherapy Department, pelvic traction can be applied more powerfully but for shorter periods. A shoulder harness is often used to give counter traction. Such traction is often efficacious for relieving pain from disc lesions even if only for a short time.

Younger more active patients can apply their own traction by stretching themselves off a bar or a strong door. Hanging by the hands for a few seconds at a time may give relief.

Distraction in extension can be applied to younger patients by the therapist standing back-to-back with the patient and linking arms. The therapist bends forwards and the patient allows himself/herself to be lifted off the ground with the lumbar spine extended. This method should be used only as a method of last resort in patients who have had a recent radiograph excluding infections and neoplasms.

Leg traction

This procedure can be applied to one or both legs to relieve unilateral or bilateral sciatica. The original intention was to stretch the lumbar spine and thus increase the height of the disc spaces with the hope of reduction of a disc prolapse. However, it is applied to patients with many varieties of low back pain from structural causes and the good effects are more likely to be the result of splinting the patient in a horizontal position in his bed. Skin traction will not support more than 4 kg on each leg (less if the leg is short or the skin is friable). It is not justified to apply skeletal traction with a trans-tibial pin for low back pain. Skin traction should not be applied if:

- The patient has a history of skin allergy
- Dermatitis is present
- Skin sepsis is present
- Heavier traction is required

Requirements for skin traction

- Razor
- Pack containing adhesive tape and spreader or rubberised tape and spreader (both commercially available)
- Spray can of tincture of benzoin compound
- Pulley bar
- Weights
- Crepe bandage

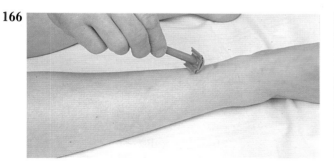

166 The leg is shaved if necessary.

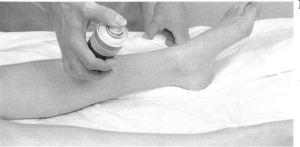

167 Tincture of benzoin compound is sprayed on the leg as an aid to adhesion.

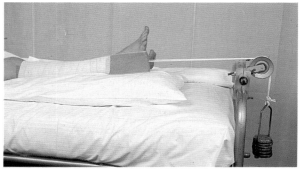

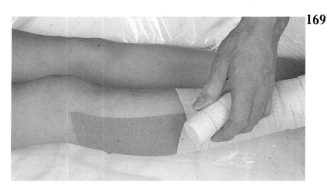

168 The adhesive tape is applied to the leg with the spreader held opposite the heel and padding against the malleoli. An assistant is an advantage.

169 The adhesive tape is secured by a crepe bandage.

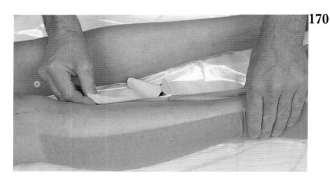

170 Skin traction completed. If heavier weights are required (up to 4 kg), additional purchase can be achieved by applying the adhesive tape to the sides of the thighs. The foot of the bed is elevated to prevent the patient being pulled down.

Pelvic traction

This is applied through a pelvic corset and a wide spreader well distal to the feet. It allows more freedom for the legs.

It can be applied if there are contraindications to skin traction on the leg(s). The maximum comfortable traction force is 10 kg through a well-fitting corset.

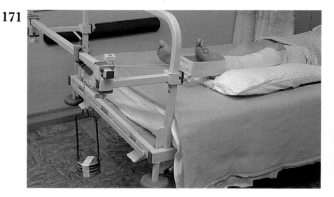

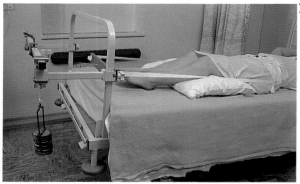

171 Leg traction should act along the line of the leg without undue elevations of the limb. A pillow under the calf and knee makes it comfortable for the patient. The end of the bed is elevated to balance the weights against the patient's bodyweight.

172 Pelvic traction complete with a wide spreader beyond the patient's feet gives freedom of leg movement. Again, the end of the bed is elevated a little.

Manipulations

This form of treatment is frequently requested and frequently applied, usually without a general anaesthetic and without previous investigation.

The minimal requirements are a full history and physical examination together with recent radiographs to exclude neoplasms and infections. The physical basis of the treatment is to stretch muscles and ligaments and to shift the facets of the posterior joints: there may be some alteration in the size and position of a disc prolapse.

Without anaesthesia the patient can resist the limits of movement imposed by the therapist, but can report the onset and distribution of pain. Most therapists aim to catch the patient unawares, so that there is no resistance to a forcible manoeuvre.

Forced passive flexion of the spine is intrinsically dangerous both with and without anaesthesia, as it can provoke a disc prolapse or a vertebral compression fracture in osteoporotic vertebrae. It should be avoided.

With general anaesthesia the lumbar spine can be quickly and gently stretched to a full range of rotation, lateral flexion and extension. Violent sudden movements and great force should not be applied. Frequently clicks and cracks are heard during manipulation. The significance of these is not known.

Indications

Acute low back pain of skeletal origin:

- Where the patient wants to mobilise or travel
- Where manipulation has been effective previously
- Where other conservative measures have failed
- Where a placebo measure seems necessary

Absolute contraindications

- Osteitis
- Osteoporosis
- Disc prolapse with neurological deficit
- Neoplasia
- Low back pain from visceral causes
- Recent surgery or chemonucleolysis

Relative contraindications

- Improving disc lesion
- Large patient, small manipulator

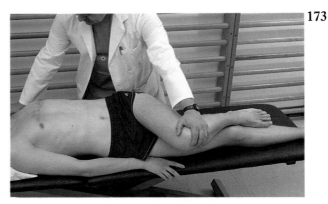
173

173 Lumbar spinal rotation. The patient lies supine and under general anaesthesia. The therapist flexes the nearest hip and knee and rotates the pelvis and lumbar spine away from him until the flexed knee touches the couch on the other side of the pelvis. The procedure is repeated from the other side of the patient.

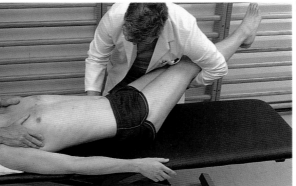
174

174 Lumbar spinal lateral flexion. The lumbar spine is flexed laterally by the therapist holding the legs and pelvis and an assistant holding the chest and shoulders.

With the patient prone the lumbar spine can be gently extended by lifting the legs and pelvis.

There are many other methods of manipulation of the lumbar spine.

Caudal epidural injections

This form of treatment aims to distend the sacral and lower lumbar spinal canal with a dilute solution of local anaesthetic agent mixed with saline i.e. 10 ml of 1 per cent lignocaine in 50 ml of normal saline. This will stretch nerve roots and adhesions almost painlessly. Some practitioners add steroids to the solution to suppress any inflammatory changes.

Indications are the failure of other forms of conservative treatment to relieve pain arising from the 4th and 5th lumbar and 1st and 2nd sacral levels.

Contraindications are infection or neoplastic change (or the suspicion thereof) in the sacral or lumbar regions.

The effects are variable but some patients obtain long-lasting relief. The injections can be repeated once or twice at weekly intervals, if only partial relief is obtained the first time.

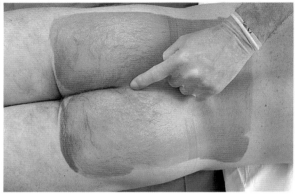

175 Caudal epidural injection is a more invasive method of treatment. The patient lies face down or on the side as for a lumbar puncture. The sacral hiatus is identified by palpation. This procedure is easier in thinner subjects and by reference to an xray.

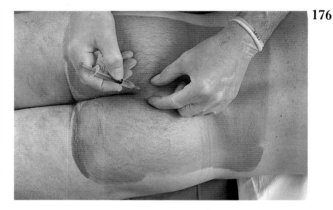

176 Local anaesthetic is injected into the overlying skin and fat.

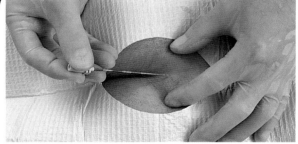

177 A long spinal needle pointing cranially is then introduced into the sacral hiatus.

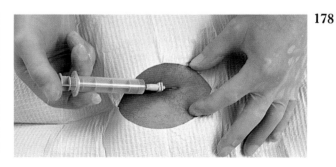

178 As the needle is pushed up the spinal canal, diluted anaesthetic solution is injected: 20-40 ml. Frequent aspirations are required to ensure there is no tap of CSF. If this occurs, no more solution is injected. Some practitioners add steroids to the diluted anaesthetic solution. The patient will experience some numbness of the perineum and buttocks for a few hours afterwards and should rest during this period.

Surgery

Chemonucleolysis

Chemonucleolysis is a technique of shrinking the nucleus pulposus by injecting a very small volume of the enzyme ananase to degrade the large molecules of glycoproteins. Good imaging and a careful technique are vital to prevent the patient becoming paraplegic. Those who have the best results are in young adult life with a central disc prolapse at one level proven by myelogram or CT scan. Symptoms from sequestrated disc material in the spinal canal cannot be relieved in this manner. Second injections may produce an allergic reaction and even first injections may lead to anaphylaxis.

The patient is heavily sedated but should be able to obey commands and respond to pain. In this state injections into the cauda equina can be avoided.

The patient is supported on a radiotranslucent mattress which allows an image intensifier to produce good quality anteroposterior and lateral views of the lumbar spine. An exact lateral posture is secured and the lumbar spine is straightened by a small pillow in the loin; 10 ml of 0.5 per cent prilocaine is injected into the loin. The needle is directed posteriorly parallel to the iliac crest.

The double-needle technique has made introduction into the centre of the disc space much easier as the malleable central needle will slide across the vertebral end plate into the nucleus pulposus. 0.5 ml of enzyme is injected and should go in with little pressure. A 60-second pause will allow monitoring by the anaesthetist to detect a rare anaphylactic response. If all is well, a further 0.5 ml is injected and the needle withdrawn.

The patient is detained in hospital for 48 hours. During this time there may be an exacerbation of back ache, but in successful cases this gradually fades over the next 6 weeks.

179

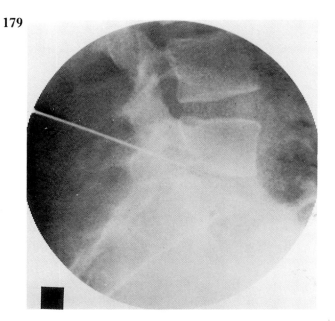

180

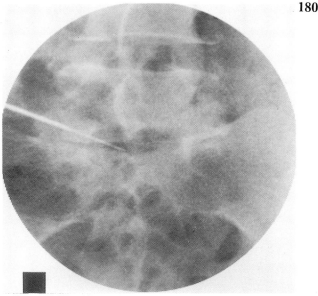

179 A lateral view of a needle entering the lumbosacral disc preparatory to chymopapein injection. The tip of the needle appears to be in a good central position but this must be confirmed by a view in the anteroposterior plane.

180 An anteroposterior view of a needle entering the lumbosacral disc before chymopapein injection. The tip of the needle is in a good position but this must be checked by a view from a lateral direction.

Structural causes

A proven prolapsed intervertebral disc causing persistent pain and/or sciatica despite conservative treatment of bedrest, weight-reduction, physiotherapy or external splintage may be enucleated by a posterior approach through the lamina of the neural arch (laminectomy or, more correctly, discectomy). In the recent past this was followed by 6 weeks' rest in bed to allow complete soft-tissue healing, but this has been found to be unnecessary; mobilisation after 2-3 days is now the rule. Percutaneous discectomy through a special arthroscope is now an experimental procedure.

In some patients with intractable sciatica, it can be shown that the lumbar or sacral nerve root is compressed by the skeletal walls of the lateral root canal and not by a prolapsed disc. Decompression of the root canal and/or excision of the neighbouring facet joint may be curative without incising the disc anteriorly.

Spondylolisthesis with intractable pain, continuing anterior displacement and an unrelieved neurological deficit may require a local one-segment spinal fusion, if a belt or a brace fail. The fusion is best performed between the vertebral bodies or between the transverse processes.

Similarly an unstable spinal vertebra caused by fracture or disc degeneration may be fused to give relief of pain. Unfortunately in all cases of surgical fusion the spinal joints above and below the fused segment are likely to undergo degenerative changes.

If surgical fusion is considered, it is important to prove by discograms, myelogram, etc. that the chief component of pain does not arise from some other structure nearby.

Neurological causes

Those few patients with a progressive neurological deficit often require urgent surgery to decompress the spinal cord, cauda equina or peripheral nerve roots.

An urgent decompressive laminectomy may allow recovery of nerves and provide biopsy material but it also has the effect of destabilising a spinal column already weakened by trauma or neoplasia. However, if a rare benign intrathecal tumour (such as a neurofibroma or neurilemmoma) is the cause of the neurological deficit, it can be removed in its entirety in many cases without destabilising the spine.

Visceral causes

These causes of low back pain are frequently amenable to surgical care, e.g. abdominal aortic aneurysm, pelvic sepsis, hydronephrosis, peptic ulceration; but neoplastic changes in the abdomen are less likely to respond completely to surgery, i.e. hypernephroma, lymphomatoma, carcinoma of the pancreas. The advice of an appropriate specialist surgeon should be sought.

181 Surgery for low back pain is confined to a small percentage (1-2 per cent) whose pain is clearly localised and whose disability has failed to respond to conservative treatment. The exceptions to this are those with incipient paraplegia or a progressive neurological deficit. The aims of surgery should be defined clearly before any action is taken and there is no place for exploratory surgery. The lesion should be located accurately, so that the surgeon knows exactly where to look and what to do.

For many operations on the lower spine the kneeling position provides good access for the surgeon and allows blood to gravitate into the abdomen or legs and not obscure the operative field. The airway and arms are easily available to the anaesthetist.

182 Bone grafts for stabilising the spine are easily obtained from the iliac crest when the muscles have been reflected.

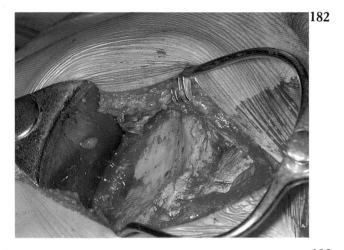

183 Bone grafts are incorporated into the recipient area if the local bone has been denuded of soft tissue and 'shingled' with an osteotome. Cancellous donor bone is incorporated better than cortical bone.

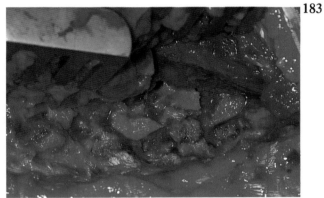

184 An anteroposterior view of the lumbar spine showing bone grafts packed between the transverse processes of L5 and the sacrum.

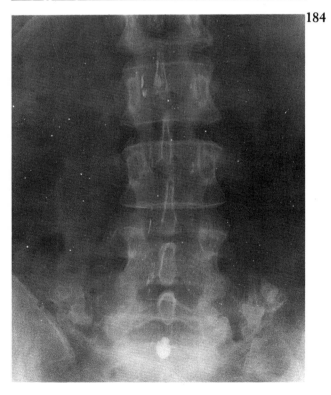

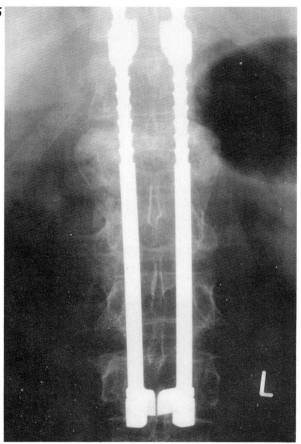

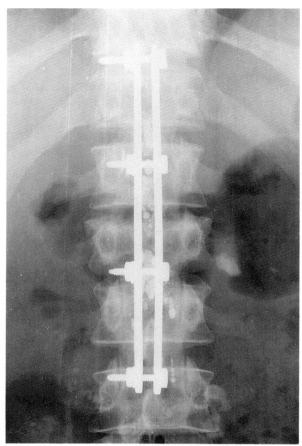

185 An anteroposterior view of the thoracolumbar spine showing a fracture at L1. There are two Harrington rods inserted to reduce and immobilise the fracture site. After union had taken place, these rods became loose and required removal.

Despite union of the fracture in a good position, degenerative changes with backache always develop at the levels immediately above and below the injury.

186 An anteroposterior view of the upper lumbar spine showing plates bolted to the spinous processes to reduce and immobilise a fracture dislocation at L1/2. This method is little used since the advent of Harrington rods.

Index

All figures refer to page numbers